FIRST AID FOR THE® PSYCHIATRY CLERKSHIP

FOURTH EDITION

LATHA GANTI, MD, MS, MBA, FACEP

Director, VACO Southeast Specialty Care
Center of Innovation
Orlando VA Medical Center
Professor of Emergency Medicine
University of Central Florida
Orlando, Florida

SEAN M. BLITZSTEIN, MD

Director, Psychiatry Clerkship
Clinical Associate Professor of Psychiatry
University of Illinois at Chicago
Chicago, Illinois

MATTHEW S. KAUFMAN, MD

Associate Director
Department of Emergency Medicine
Richmond University Medical Center
New York, New York

McGraw Hill Education

New York / Chicago / San Francisco / Athens / Lisbon / London / Madrid / Mexico City
Milan / New Delhi / Singapore / Sydney / Toronto

First Aid for the® Psychiatry Clerkship, Fourth Edition

2 3 4 5 6 7 8 9 0   ROV/ROV   20 19 18 17 16

ISBN 978-0-07-184174-0
MHID 0-07-184174-1

Notice

Medicine is an ever-changing science. As new research and clinical experience broaden our knowledge, changes in treatment and drug therapy are required. The authors and the publisher of this work have checked with sources believed to be reliable in their efforts to provide information that is complete and generally in accord with the standards accepted at the time of publication. However, in view of the possibility of human error or changes in medical sciences, neither the authors nor the publisher nor any other party who has been involved in the preparation or publication of this work warrants that the information contained herein is in every respect accurate or complete, and they disclaim all responsibility for any errors or omissions or for the results obtained from use of the information contained in this work. Readers are encouraged to confirm the information contained herein with other sources. For example and in particular, readers are advised to check the product information sheet included in the package of each drug they plan to administer to be certain that the information contained in this work is accurate and that changes have not been made in the recommended dose or in the contraindications for administration. This recommendation is of particular importance in connection with new or infrequently used drugs.

This book was set in Electra LT Std Regular by MPS Limited.
The editors were Catherine A. Johnson and Christina M. Thomas.
The production supervisor was Catherine Saggese.
Project management was provided by Asheesh Ratra, MPS Limited.
RR Donnelley/Owensville was printer and binder.

This book is printed on acid-free paper.

Library of Congress Cataloging-in-Publication Data

Ganti, Latha, author.
    First aid for the psychiatry clerkship / Latha Ganti, Matthew S. Kaufman. — Fourth edition.
        p. ; cm.
    Includes index.
    ISBN 978-0-07-184174-0 (pbk. : alk. paper) — ISBN 0-07-184174-1
    I. Kaufman, Matthew S., author.   II. Title.
    [DNLM: 1. Mental Disorders—Outlines.   2. Clinical Clerkship—Outlines.
3. Psychiatry—Outlines. WM 18.2]
    RC480.5
    616.890071—dc23
                                                                    2015029130

International Edition ISBN 978-1-259-25118-4; MHID 1-259-25118-7. Copyright © 2016 by McGraw-Hill Education. Exclusive rights by McGraw-Hill Education for manufacture and export. This book cannot be re-exported from the country to which it is consigned by McGraw-Hill Education. The International Edition is not available in North America.

McGraw-Hill Education books are available at special quantity discounts to use as premiums and sales promotions, or for use in corporate training programs. To contact a representative please visit the Contact Us pages at www.mhprofessional.com.

CONTENTS

Contributing Authors   v

Introduction   vii

Chapter 1:   How to Succeed in the Psychiatry Clerkship   1

Chapter 2:   Examination and Diagnosis   11

Chapter 3:   Psychotic Disorders   21

Chapter 4:   Mood Disorders   33

Chapter 5:   Anxiety, Obsessive-Compulsive, Trauma, and Stressor-Related Disorders   47

Chapter 6:   Personality Disorders   63

Chapter 7:   Substance-Related and Addictive Disorders   79

Chapter 8:   Neurocognitive Disorders   97

Chapter 9:   Geriatric Psychiatry   113

Chapter 10: Psychiatric Disorders in Children   121

Chapter 11: Dissociative Disorders   133

Chapter 12: Somatic Symptom and Factitious Disorders   139

Chapter 13: Impulse Control Disorders   145

Chapter 14: Eating Disorders   151

Chapter 15: Sleep-Wake Disorders   159

Chapter 16: Sexual Dysfunctions and Paraphilic Disorders   171

Chapter 17: Psychotherapies   179

Chapter 18: Psychopharmacology   189

Chapter 19: Forensic Psychiatry   209

Index   217

CONTRIBUTING AUTHORS

SEAN M. BLITZSTEIN, MD

Director, Psychiatry Clerkship
Clinical Associate Professor of Psychiatry
University of Illinois at Chicago
Chicago, Illinois
Examination and Diagnosis
Personality Disorders
Substance-Related and Addictive Disorders
Geriatric Psychiatry
Somatic Symptom and Factitious Disorders
Sexual Dysfunctions and Paraphilic Disorders

AMBER C. MAY, MD

Resident, Department of Psychiatry
University of Illinois at Chicago
Chicago, Illinois
Anxiety, Obsessive-Compulsive, Trauma and Stressor-Related Disorders
Neurocognitive Disorders
Psychiatric Disorders in Children
Dissociative Disorders

KELLEY A. VOLPE, MD

Chief Resident, Department of Psychiatry
University of Illinois at Chicago College of Medicine
Chicago, Illinois
Eating Disorders
Sleep-Wake Disorders
Psychotherapies
Forensic Psychiatry

ALEXANDER YUEN, MD

Resident, Department of Psychiatry
University of Illinois at Chicago
Chicago, Illinois
Psychotic Disorders
Mood Disorders
Impulse Control Disorders
Psychopharmacology

INTRODUCTION

This clinical study aid was designed in the tradition of the First Aid series of books. It is formatted in the same way as the other books in this series; however, a stronger clinical emphasis was placed on its content in relation to psychiatry. You will find that rather than simply preparing you for success on the clerkship exam, this resource will help guide you in the clinical diagnosis and treatment of many problems seen by psychiatrists.

Each of the chapters in this book contains the major topics central to the practice of psychiatry and has been specifically designed for the medical student learning level. It contains information that psychiatry clerks are expected to learn and will ultimately be responsible for on their shelf exams.

The content of the text is organized in the format similar to other texts in the First Aid series. Topics are listed by bold headings, and the "meat" of the topics provides essential information. The outside margins contain mnemonics, diagrams, exam and ward tips, summary or warning statements, and other memory aids. Exam tips are marked by the 🔑 icon, tips for the wards by the 🖐 icon, and clinical scenarios by the 🧍 icon.

CHAPTER 1

HOW TO SUCCEED IN THE PSYCHIATRY CLERKSHIP

Why Spend Time on Psychiatry?	2	Keep Patient Information Handy	3
How to Behave on the Wards	2	Present Patient Information in an Organized Manner	3
Respect the Patients	2	How to Prepare for the Clerkship (Shelf) Exam	4
Respect the Field of Psychiatry	2	Study with Friends	4
Take Responsibility for Your Patients	3	Study in a Bright Room	4
Respect Patients' Rights	3	Eat Light, Balanced Meals	4
Volunteer	3	Take Practice Exams	4
Be a Team Player	3	Pocket Cards	5

The psychiatry clerkship will most likely be very interesting and exciting.

A key to doing well in this clerkship is finding the balance between drawing a firm boundary of professionalism with your patients and creating a relationship of trust and comfort.

Why Spend Time on Psychiatry?

For most, your medical school psychiatry clerkship will encompass the entirety of your formal training in psychiatry during your career in medicine.

Being aware of and understanding the features of mental dysfunction in psychiatric patients will serve you well in recognizing psychiatric symptoms in your patients, regardless of your specialty choice.

While anxiety and depression can worsen the prognosis of patients' other medical conditions, medical illnesses can cause significant psychological stress, often uncovering a previously subclinical psychiatric condition. The stress of extended hospitalizations can strain normal mental and emotional functioning beyond their adaptive reserve, resulting in transient psychiatric symptoms.

Psychotropic medications are frequently prescribed in the general population. Many of these drugs have significant medical side effects and drug interactions. You will become familiar with these during your clerkship and will encounter them in clinical practice regardless of your field of medicine.

Because of the unique opportunity to spend a great deal of time interacting with your patients, the psychiatry clerkship is an excellent time to practice your interview skills and "bedside manner."

How to Behave on the Wards

RESPECT THE PATIENTS

Always maintain professionalism and show the patients respect. Be respectful when discussing cases with your residents and attendings.

RESPECT THE FIELD OF PSYCHIATRY

- Regardless of your interest in psychiatry, take the rotation seriously.
- You may not agree with all the decisions that your residents and attendings make, but it is important for everyone to be on the same page. Be aware of patients who try to split you from your team.
- Dress in a professional, conservative manner.
- Working with psychiatric patients can often be emotionally taxing. Keep yourself healthy.
- Psychiatry is a multidisciplinary field. It would behoove you to continuously communicate with nurses, social workers, and psychologists.
- Address patients formally unless otherwise told.

TAKE RESPONSIBILITY FOR YOUR PATIENTS

Know as much as possible about your patients: their history, psychiatric and medical problems, test results, treatment plan, and prognosis. Keep your intern or resident informed of new developments that they might not be aware of, and ask them for any updates you might not be aware of. Assist the team in developing a plan; speak to consultants and family members. Never deliver bad news to patients or family members without the assistance of your supervising resident or attending.

RESPECT PATIENTS' RIGHTS

1. All patients have the right to have their personal medical information kept private. This means do not discuss the patient's information with family members without that patient's consent, and do not discuss any patient in public areas (e.g., hallways, elevators, cafeterias).
2. All patients have the right to refuse treatment. This means they can refuse treatment by a specific individual (the medical student) or of a specific type (no electroconvulsive therapy). Patients can even refuse lifesaving treatment. The only exceptions to this rule are if the patient is deemed to not have the capacity to make decisions or if the patient is suicidal or homicidal.
3. All patients should be informed of the right to seek advance directives on admission. Often, this is done by the admissions staff or by a social worker. If your patient is chronically ill or has a life-threatening illness, address the subject of advance directives with the assistance of your resident or attending.

VOLUNTEER

Be enthusiastic and self-motivated. Volunteer to help with a procedure or a difficult task. Volunteer to give a 20-minute talk on a topic of your choice, to take additional patients, and to stay late.

BE A TEAM PLAYER

Help other medical students with their tasks; teach them information you have learned. Support your supervising intern or resident whenever possible. Never steal the spotlight or make a fellow medical student look bad.

KEEP PATIENT INFORMATION HANDY

Use a clipboard, notebook, or index cards to keep patient information, including a history and physical, lab, and test results, at hand.

PRESENT PATIENT INFORMATION IN AN ORGANIZED MANNER

Here is a template for the "bullet" presentation:

"This is a [age]-year-old [gender] with a history of [major history such as bipolar disorder] who presented on [date] with [major symptoms, such as auditory hallucinations] and was found to have [working diagnosis]. [Tests done] showed [results]. Yesterday, the patient [state important changes, new plan, new tests, new medications]. This morning the patient feels [state the patient's words], and the mental status and physical exams are significant for [state major findings]. Plan is [state plan]."

The newly admitted patient generally deserves a longer presentation following the complete history and physical format.

Many patients have extensive histories. The complete history should be present in the admission note, but during ward presentations, the entire history is often too much to absorb. In these cases, it will be very important that you generate a **good summary** that is concise but maintains an accurate picture of the patient.

How to Prepare for the Clerkship (Shelf) Exam

If you have studied the core psychiatric symptoms and illnesses, you will know a great deal about psychiatry. To specifically study for the clerkship or shelf exam, we recommend:

2–3 weeks before exam: Read this entire review book, taking notes.
10 days before exam: Read the notes you took during the rotation and the corresponding review book sections.
5 days before exam: Read this entire review book, concentrating on lists and mnemonics.
2 days before exam: Exercise, eat well, skim the book, and go to bed early.
1 day before exam: Exercise, eat well, review your notes and the mnemonics, and go to bed on time. Do not have any caffeine after 2 PM.

Other helpful studying strategies include:

STUDY WITH FRIENDS

Group studying can be very helpful. Other people may point out areas that you have not studied enough and may help you focus more effectively. If you tend to get distracted by other people in the room, limit this amount to less than half of your study time.

STUDY IN A BRIGHT ROOM

Find the room in your home or library that has the brightest light. This will help prevent you from falling asleep. If you don't have a bright light, obtain a halogen desk lamp or a light that simulates sunlight.

EAT LIGHT, BALANCED MEALS

Make sure your meals are balanced, with lean protein, fruits and vegetables, and fiber. A high-sugar, high-carbohydrate meal will give you an initial burst of energy for 1–2 hours, but then your blood sugar will quickly drop.

TAKE PRACTICE EXAMS

The purpose of practice exams is not just for the content that is contained in the questions, but the process of sitting for several hours and attempting to choose the best answer for each and every question.

POCKET CARDS

The "cards" on the following page contain information that is often helpful in psychiatry practice. We advise that you make a photocopy of these cards, cut them out, and carry them in your coat pocket.

Mental Status Exam

Appearance/Behavior: apparent age, attitude and cooperativeness, eye contact, posture, dress and hygiene, psychomotor status

Speech: rate, rhythm, volume, tone, articulation

Mood: patient's subjective emotional state—depressed, anxious, sad, angry, etc.

Affect: objective emotional expression—euthymic, dysphoric, euphoric, appropriate (to stated mood), labile, full, constricted, flat, etc.

Thought process: logical/linear, circumstantial, tangential, flight of ideas, looseness of association, thought blocking

Thought content: suicidal/homicidal ideation, delusions, preoccupations, hyperreligiosity

Perceptual disturbances: hallucinations, illusions, derealization, depersonalization

Cognition:
  Level of consciousness: alert, sleepy, lethargic
  Orientation: person, place, date
  Attention/concentration: serial 7s, spell "world" backwards

Memory:
  Registration: immediate recall of three objects
  Short term: recall of objects after 5 minutes
  Long term: ask about verifiable personal information

Fund of knowledge: current events

Abstract thought: interpretation of proverbs, analogies

Insight: patient's awareness of his/her illness and need for treatment

Judgment: patient's ability to approach his/her problems in an appropriate manner

Delirium

Characteristics: acute onset, waxing/waning sensorium (worse at night), disorientation, inattention, impaired cognition, disorganized thinking, altered sleep-wake cycle, perceptual disorders (hallucinations, illusions)

(continued)

Etiology: drugs (narcotics, benzodiazepines, anticholinergics, TCAs, steroids, diphenhydramine, etc.), EtOH withdrawal, metabolic (cardiac, respiratory, renal, hepatic, endocrine), infection, neurological causes (increased ICP, encephalitis, postictal, stroke)

Investigations:

Routine: CBC, electrolytes, glucose, renal panel, LFTs, TFTs, UA, urine toxicology, CXR, O_2 sat, HIV
Medium-yield: ABG, ECG (silent MI), ionized Ca^{2+}
If above inconclusive: Head CT/MRI, EEG, LP

Management: identify/correct underlying cause, simplify Rx regimen, d/c potentially offensive medications if possible, avoid benzodiazepines (except in EtOH withdrawal), create safe environment, provide reassurance/education, judiciously use antipsychotics for acute agitation

---

Mini-Mental State Examination (MMSE)

Orientation (10):

What is the [year] [season] [date] [day] [month]? (1 pt. each)
Where are we [state] [county] [town] [hospital] [floor]?

Registration (3): Ask the patient to repeat three unrelated objects (1 pt. each on first attempt). If incomplete on first attempt, repeat up to six times (record # of trials).

Attention (5): Either serial 7s or "world" backwards (1 pt. for each correct letter or number).

Delayed recall (3): Ask patient to recall the three objects previously named (1 pt. each).

Language (9):

- Name two common objects, e.g., watch, pen (1 pt. each).
- Repeat the following sentence: "No ifs, ands, or buts" (1 pt.).
- Give patient blank paper. "Take it in your right hand, use both hands to fold it in half, and then put it on the floor" (1 pt. for each part correctly executed).
- Have patient read and follow: "Close your eyes" (1 pt.).
- Ask patient to write a sentence. The sentence must contain a subject and a verb; correct grammar and punctuation are not necessary (1 pt.)
- Ask the patient to copy the design. Each figure must have five sides, and two of the angles must intersect (1 pt.).

Mania ("DIG FAST")

Distractibility
Irritable mood/insomnia
Grandiosity
Flight of ideas
Agitation/increase in goal-directed activity
Speedy thoughts/speech
Thoughtlessness: seek pleasure without regard to consequences

Suicide Risk ("SAD PERSONS")

Sex—male
Age >60 years
Depression
Previous attempt
Ethanol/drug abuse
Rational thinking loss
Suicide in family
Organized plan/access
No support
Sickness

Depression ("SIG E. CAPS")

Sleep
Interest
Guilt
Energy
Concentration
Appetite
Psychomotor Δs
Suicidal ideation
   Hopelessness
   Helplessness
   Worthlessness

Drugs of Abuse

Drug	Intoxication	Withdrawal
Alcohol Benzodiazepines	Disinhibition, mood lability, incoordination, slurred speech, ataxia, blackouts (EtOH), respiratory depression	Tremulousness, hypertension, tachycardia, anxiety, psychomotor agitation, nausea, seizures, hallucinations, DTs (EtOH)
Barbiturates	Respiratory depression	Anxiety, seizures, delirium, life-threatening cardiovascular collapse

(continued)

Opioids	CNS depression, nausea, vomiting, sedation, decreased pain perception, decreased GI motility, pupil constriction, respiratory depression	Increased sympathetic activity, N/V, diarrhea, diaphoresis, rhinorrhea, piloerection, yawning, stomach cramps, myalgias, arthralgias, restlessness, anxiety, anorexia
Amphetamines Cocaine	Euphoria, increased attention span, aggressiveness, psychomotor agitation, pupil dilatation, hypertension, tachycardia, cardiac arrhythmias, psychosis (paranoia with amphetamines, formication with cocaine)	Post-use "crash": restlessness, headache, hunger, severe depression, irritability, insomnia/ hypersomnia, strong psychological craving
PCP	Belligerence, impulsiveness, psychomotor agitation, vertical/horizontal nystagmus, hyperthermia, tachycardia, ataxia, psychosis, homicidality	May have recurrence of symptoms due to reabsorption in GI tract
LSD	Altered perceptual states (hallucinations, distortions of time and space), elevation of mood, "bad trips" (panic reaction), flashbacks (reexperience of the sensations in absence of drug use)	
Cannabis	Euphoria, anxiety, paranoia, slowed time, social withdrawal, increased appetite, dry mouth, tachycardia, amotivational syndrome	
Nicotine/ Caffeine	Restlessness, insomnia, anxiety, anorexia	Irritability, lethargy, headache, increased appetite, weight gain

Psychiatric Emergencies

Delirium Tremens (DTs):

- Typically within 2–4 days after cessation of EtOH but may occur later.
- Delirium, agitation, fever, autonomic hyperactivity, auditory and visual hallucinations.
- Treat aggressively with benzodiazepines and hydration.

Neuroleptic Malignant Syndrome (NMS):

- Fever, rigidity, autonomic instability, clouding of consciousness, elevated WBC/CPK
- Withhold neuroleptics, hydrate, consider dantrolene and/or bromocriptine
- Idiosyncratic, time-limited reaction

Serotonin Syndrome:

- Precipitated by use of two drugs with serotonin-enhancing properties (e.g., MAOI + SSRI).
- Altered mental status, fever, agitation, tremor, myoclonus, hyperreflexia, ataxia, incoordination, diaphoresis, shivering, diarrhea.
- Discontinue offending agents, benzodiazepines, consider cyproheptadine.

Tyramine Reaction/Hypertensive Crisis:

- Precipitated by ingestion of tyramine containing foods while on MAOIs.
- Hypertension, headache, neck stiffness, sweating, nausea, vomiting, visual problems. Most serious consequences are stroke and possibly death.
- Treat with nitroprusside or phentolamine.

Acute Dystonia:

- Early, sudden onset of muscle spasm: eyes, tongue, jaw, neck; may lead to laryngospasm requiring intubation.
- Treat with benztropine (Cogentin) or diphenhydramine (Benadryl).

Lithium Toxicity:

- May occur at any Li level (usually >1.5).
- Nausea, vomiting, slurred speech, ataxia, incoordination, myoclonus, hyperreflexia, seizures, nephrogenic diabetes insipidus, delirium, coma
- Discontinue Li, hydrate aggressively, consider hemodialysis

Tricyclic Antidepressant (TCA) Toxicity:

- Primarily anticholinergic effects; cardiac conduction disturbances, hypotension, respiratory depression, agitation, hallucinations.
- CNS stimulation, depression, seizures.
- Monitor ECG, activated charcoal, cathartics, supportive treatment.

NOTES

CHAPTER 2

EXAMINATION AND DIAGNOSIS

History and Mental Status Examination   12

    INTERVIEWING   12

    TAKING THE HISTORY   13

    MENTAL STATUS EXAMINATION   14

    MINI-MENTAL STATE EXAMINATION (MMSE)   17

Interviewing Skills   17

    GENERAL APPROACHES TO TYPES OF PATIENTS   17

Diagnosis and Classification   18

    DIAGNOSIS AS PER DSM-5   18

Diagnostic Testing   18

    INTELLIGENCE TESTS   18

    OBJECTIVE PERSONALITY ASSESSMENT TESTS   19

    PROJECTIVE (PERSONALITY) ASSESSMENT TESTS   19

History and Mental Status Examination

INTERVIEWING

Making the Patient Comfortable

The initial interview is of utmost importance to the psychiatrist. With practice, you will develop your own style and learn how to adapt the interview to the individual patient. In general, start the interview by asking open-ended questions and carefully note how the patient responds, as this is critical information for the mental status exam. Consider preparing for the interview by writing down the subheadings of the exam (see Figure 2-1). Find a safe and private area to conduct the interview. Use closed-ended questions to obtain the remaining pertinent information. During the first interview, the psychiatrist

WARDS TIP

The HPI should include information about the current episode, including symptoms, duration, context, stressors, and impairment in function.

Date and Location:

Identifying Patient Data:

Chief Complaint: Past Medical History:

History of Present Illness:

                                        Allergies:

Past Psychiatric History: Current Meds:

First contact:

Diagnosis: Developmental History:

Prior hospitalizations:

Suicide attempts: Relationships (children/marital status):

Outpatient treatment:

                                      Education:

Med trials: Work History:

Substance History: Military History:

                                      Housing:

Smoking: Income:

Family Psychiatric History: Religion:

Legal History:

FIGURE 2-1. **Psychiatric history outline.**

must establish a meaningful rapport with the patient in order to get accurate and pertinent information. This requires that questions be asked in a quiet, comfortable setting so that the patient is at ease. The patient should feel that the psychiatrist is interested, nonjudgmental, and compassionate. In psychiatry, the history is the most important factor in formulating a diagnosis and treatment plan.

TAKING THE HISTORY

The psychiatric history follows a similar format as the history for other types of patients. It should include the following:

- Identifying data: The patient's name, gender, age, race, marital status, place and type of residence, occupation.
- Chief complaint (use the patient's own words). If called as a consultant, list reason for the consult.
- Sources of information.
- History of present illness (HPI):
  - *The 4 Ps*: The patient's psychosocial and environmental conditions *predisposing to, precipitating, perpetuating,* and *protecting* against the current episode.
  - The patient's support system (whom the patient lives with, distance and level of contact with friends and relatives).
  - Neurovegetative symptoms (quality of sleep, appetite, energy, psychomotor retardation/activation, concentration).
  - Suicidal ideation/homicidal ideation.
  - How work and relationship have been affected (for most diagnoses in the *Diagnostic and Statistical Manual of Mental Disorders*, 5th edition [DSM-5] there is a criterion that specifies that symptoms must cause clinically significant distress or impairment in social, occupational, or other important areas of functioning).
  - Psychotic symptoms (e.g., auditory and visual hallucinations).
  - Establish a baseline of mental health:
    - Patient's level of functioning when "well"
    - Goals (outpatient setting)
- Past psychiatric history (include as applicable: history of suicide attempts, history of self-harm [e.g., cutting, burning oneself], information about previous episodes, other psychiatric disorders in remission, medication trials, past psychiatric hospitalizations, current psychiatrist).
- Substance history (history of intravenous drug use, participation in outpatient or inpatient drug rehab programs).
- Medical history (ask specifically about head trauma, seizures, pregnancy status).
- Family psychiatric and medical history (include suicides and treatment response as patient may respond similarly).
- Medications (ask about supplements and over-the-counter medications).
- Allergies: Clarify if it was a true allergy or an adverse drug event (e.g., abdominal pain).
- Developmental history: Achieved developmental milestones on time, friends in school, performance academically.
- Social history: Include income source, employment, education, place of residence, who they live with, number of children, support system, religious affiliation and beliefs, legal history, amount of exercise, history of trauma or abuse.

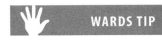

WARDS TIP

If you are seeing the patient in the ER, make sure to ask how they got to the ER (police, bus, walk-in, family member) and look to see what time they were triaged. For all initial evaluations, ask why the patient is seeking treatment *today* as opposed to any other day.

WARDS TIP

When taking a substance history, remember to ask about caffeine and nicotine use. If a heavy smoker is hospitalized and does not have access to nicotine replacement therapy, nicotine withdrawal may cause anxiety and agitation.

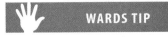

KEY FACT

Importance of asking about OTC use: Nonsteroidal anti-inflammatory drugs (NSAIDs) can ↓ lithium excretion → ↑ lithium concentrations (exceptions may be sulindac and aspirin).

WARDS TIP

Psychomotor retardation, which refers to the slowness of voluntary and involuntary movements, may also be referred to as hypokinesia or bradykinesia. The term akinesia is used in extreme cases where absence of movement is observed.

KEY FACT

Automatisms are spontaneous, involuntary movements that occur during an altered state of consciousness and can range from purposeful to disorganized.

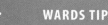

MENTAL STATUS EXAMINATION

This is analogous to performing a physical exam in other areas of medicine. It is the nuts and bolts of the psychiatric exam. It should describe the patient in as much detail as possible. The mental status exam assesses the following:

- Appearance
- Behavior
- Speech
- Mood/Affect
- Thought Process
- Thought Content
- Perceptual Disturbances
- Cognition
- Insight
- Judgment/Impulse Control

The mental status exam tells only about the mental status at that moment; it can change every hour or every day, etc.

Appearance/Behavior

- *Physical appearance:* Gender, age (looks older/younger than stated age), type of clothing, hygiene (including smelling of alcohol, urine, feces), posture, grooming, physical abnormalities, tattoos, body piercings. Take specific notice of the following, which may be clues for possible diagnoses:
  - Pupil size: Drug intoxication/withdrawal.
  - Bruises in hidden areas: ↑ suspicion for abuse.
  - Needle marks/tracks: Drug use.
  - Eroding of tooth enamel: Eating disorders (from vomiting).
  - Superficial cuts on arms: Self-harm.
- *Behavior and psychomotor activity:* Attitude (cooperative, seductive, flattering, charming, eager to please, entitled, controlling, uncooperative, hostile, guarded, critical, antagonistic, childish), mannerisms, tics, eye contact, activity level, psychomotor retardation/activation, akathisia, automatisms, catatonia, choreoathetoid movements, compulsions, dystonias, tremor.

Speech

Rate (pressured, slowed, regular), rhythm (i.e., prosody), articulation (dysarthria, stuttering), accent/dialect, volume/modulation (loudness or softness), tone, long or short latency of speech.

Mood

Mood is the emotion that the patient tells you he feels, often in quotations.

Affect

Affect is an assessment of how the patient's mood appears to the examiner, including the amount and range of emotional expression. It is described with the following dimensions:

- *Type of affect:* Euthymic, euphoric, neutral, dysphoric.
- *Quality/Range* describes the depth and range of the feelings shown. Parameters: flat (none)—blunted (shallow)—constricted (limited)—full (average)—intense (more than normal).
- *Motility* describes how quickly a person appears to shift emotional states. Parameters: sluggish—supple—labile.

Appropriateness to content describes whether the affect is congruent with the subject of conversation or stated mood. Parameters: appropriate—not appropriate.

Thought Process

The patient's form of thinking—how he or she uses language and puts ideas together. It describes whether the patient's thoughts are logical, meaningful, and goal directed. It does not comment on *what* the patient thinks, only *how* the patient expresses his or her thoughts. **Circumstantiality** is when the point of the conversation is eventually reached but with overinclusion of trivial or irrelevant details. Examples of thought disorders include:

- **Tangentiality:** Point of conversation never reached; responses usually in the ballpark.
- **Loosening of associations:** No logical connection from one thought to another.
- **Flight of ideas:** Thoughts change abruptly from one idea to another, usually accompanied by rapid/pressured speech.
- **Neologisms:** Made-up words.
- **Word salad:** Incoherent collection of words.
- **Clang associations:** Word connections due to phonetics rather than actual meaning. "My car is red. I've been in bed. It hurts my head."
- **Thought blocking:** Abrupt cessation of communication before the idea is finished.

Thought Content

Describes the types of ideas expressed by the patient. Examples of disorders:

- **Poverty of thought versus overabundance:** Too few versus too many ideas expressed.
- **Delusions:** Fixed, false beliefs that are not shared by the person's culture and cannot be changed by reasoning. Delusions are classified as bizarre (impossible to be true) or nonbizarre (at least possible).
- **Suicidal and homicidal ideation:** Ask if the patient feels like harming him/herself or others. Identify if the plan is well formulated. Ask if the patient has an intent (i.e., if released right now, would he go and kill himself or harm others?). Ask if the patient has means to kill himself (firearms in the house/multiple prescription bottles).
- **Phobias:** Persistent, irrational fears.
- **Obsessions:** Repetitive, intrusive thoughts.
- **Compulsions:** Repetitive behaviors (usually linked with obsessive thoughts).

Perceptual Disturbances

- *Hallucinations:* Sensory perceptions that occur in the absence of an actual stimulus.
  - Describe the sensory modality: Auditory (most common), visual, taste, olfactory, or tactile.
  - Describe the details (e.g., auditory hallucinations may be ringing, humming, whispers, or voices speaking clear words). Command auditory hallucinations are voices that instruct the patient to do something.
  - Ask if the hallucination is experienced only before falling asleep (hypnagogic hallucination) or upon awakening (hypnopompic hallucination).

- *Illusions:* Inaccurate perception of existing sensory stimuli (e.g., wall appears as if it's moving).
- *Derealization/Depersonalization:* The experience of feeling detached from one's surroundings/mental processes.

Sensorium and Cognition

Sensorium and cognition are assessed in the following ways:

- **Consciousness:** Patient's level of awareness; possible range includes: Alert—drowsy—lethargic—stuporous—coma.
- **Orientation:** To person, place, and time.
- **Calculation:** Ability to add/subtract.
- **Memory:**
  - Immediate (registration)—dependent on attention/concentration and can be tested by asking a patient to repeat several digits or words.
  - Recent (short-term memory)—events within the past few minutes, hours or days.
  - Remote memory (long-term memory).
- **Fund of knowledge:** Level of knowledge in the context of the patient's culture and education (e.g., Who is the president? Who was Picasso?).
- **Attention/Concentration:** Ability to subtract serial 7s from 100 or to spell "world" backwards.
- **Reading/Writing:** Simple sentences (must make sure the patient is literate first).
- **Abstract concepts:** Ability to explain similarities between objects and understand the meaning of simple proverbs.

Insight

Insight is the patient's level of awareness and understanding of his or her problem. Problems with insight include complete denial of illness or blaming it on something else. Insight can be described as full, partial/limited, or none.

Judgment

Judgment is the patient's ability to understand the outcome of his or her actions and use this awareness in decision making. Best determined from information from the HPI and recent behavior (e.g., how a patient was brought to treatment or medication compliance). Judgment can be described as excellent, good, fair, or poor.

Mrs. Gong is a 52-year-old Asian-American woman who arrives at the emergency room reporting that her deceased husband of 25 years told her that he would be waiting for her there. In order to meet him, she drove nonstop for 22 hours from a nearby state. She claims that her husband is a famous preacher and that she, too, has a mission from God. Although she does not specify the details of her mission, she says that she was given the ability to stop time until her mission is completed. She reports experiencing high levels of energy despite not sleeping for 22 hours. She also reports that she has a history of psychiatric hospitalizations but refuses to provide further information.

While obtaining her history you perform a mental status exam. Her **appearance** is that of a woman who looks older than her stated age. She is obese and unkempt. There is no evidence of tattoos or piercings. She has tousled hair and is dressed in a mismatched flowered skirt and

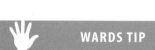
WARDS TIP

Alcoholic hallucinosis refers to hallucinations (usually auditory, although visual and tactile may occur) that occur either during or after a period of heavy alcohol consumption. Patients usually are aware that these hallucinations are not real. In contrast to delirium tremens (DTs), there is no clouding of sensorium and vital signs are normal.

a red T-shirt. Upon her arrival at the emergency room, her **behavior** is demanding, as she insists that you let her husband know that she has arrived. She then becomes irate and proceeds to yell, banging her head against the wall. She screams, "Stop hiding him from me!" She is uncooperative with redirection and is guarded during the remainder of the interview. Her eye contact is poor as she is looking around the room. Her **psychomotor activity** is agitated. Her **speech** is loud and pressured, with a foreign accent.

She reports that her **mood** is "angry," and her **affect** as observed during the interview is labile and irritable.

Her **thought process** includes flight of ideas. Her **thought content** is significant for delusions of grandeur and thought broadcasting, as evidenced by her refusing to answer most questions claiming that you are able to know what she is thinking. She denies suicidal or homicidal ideation. She expresses **disturbances in perception** as she admits to frequent auditory hallucinations of command.

She is uncooperative with formal **cognitive** testing, but you notice that she is oriented to place and person. However, she erroneously states that it is 2005. Her attention and concentration are notably impaired, as she appears distracted and frequently needs questions repeated. Her **insight, judgment, and impulse control** are determined to be poor.

You decide to admit Mrs. Gong to the inpatient psychiatric unit in order to allow for comprehensive diagnostic evaluation, the opportunity to obtain collateral information from her prior hospitalizations, safety monitoring, medical workup for possible reversible causes of her symptoms, and psychopharmacological treatment.

MINI-MENTAL STATE EXAMINATION (MMSE)

The MMSE is a simple, brief test used to assess gross cognitive functioning. See the Cognitive Disorders chapter for detailed description. The areas tested include:

- Orientation (to person, place, and time).
- Memory (immediate—registering three words; and recent—recalling three words 5 minutes later).
- Concentration and attention (serial 7s, spell "world" backwards).
- Language (naming, repetition, comprehension).
- Complex command.
- Visuospatial ability (copy of design).

Interviewing Skills

GENERAL APPROACHES TO TYPES OF PATIENTS

Violent Patient

One should avoid being alone with a potentially violent patient. Inform staff of your whereabouts. Know if there are accessible panic buttons. To assess violence or homicidality, one can simply ask, "Do you feel like you

To test ability to abstract, ask:
1. Similarities: How are an apple and orange alike? (Normal answer: "They are fruits." *Concrete* answer: "They are round.")
2. Proverb testing: What is meant by the phrase, "You can't judge a book by its cover?" (Normal answer: "You can't judge people just by how they look." *Concrete* answer: "Books have different covers.")

A prior history of violence is the most important predictor of future violence.

In assessing suicidality, do not simply ask, "Do you want to hurt yourself?" because this does not directly address suicidality (he may plan on dying in a painless way). Ask directly about killing self or suicide. If contemplating suicide, ask the patient if he has a plan of how to do it and if he has intent; a detailed plan, intent, and the means to accomplish it suggest a serious threat.

The Minnesota Multiphasic Personality Inventory (MMPI) is an objective psychological test that is used to assess a person's personality and identify psychopathologies. The mean score for each scale is 50 and the standard deviation is 10.

want to hurt someone or that you might hurt someone?" If the patient expresses imminent threats against friends, family, or others, the doctor should notify potential victims and/or protection agencies when appropriate (Tarasoff rule).

Delusional Patient

Although the psychiatrist should not directly challenge a delusion or insist that it is untrue, he should not imply he believes it either. He should simply acknowledge that he understands the *patient believes* the delusion is true.

Depressed Patient

A depressed patient may be skeptical that he or she can be helped. It is important to offer reassurance that he or she can improve with appropriate therapy. Inquiring about suicidal thoughts is crucial; a feeling of hopelessness, substance use, and/or a history of prior suicide attempts reveal an ↑ risk for suicide. If the patient is actively planning or contemplating suicide, he or she should be hospitalized or otherwise protected.

Diagnosis and Classification

DIAGNOSIS AS PER DSM-5

The American Psychiatric Association uses a criterion-based system for diagnoses. Criteria and codes for each diagnosis are outlined in the DSM-5.

Diagnostic Testing

INTELLIGENCE TESTS

Aspects of intelligence include memory, logical reasoning, ability to assimilate factual knowledge, understanding of abstract concepts, etc.

Intelligence Quotient (IQ)

IQ is a test of intelligence with a mean of 100 and a standard deviation of 15. These scores are adjusted for age. An IQ of 100 signifies that mental age equals chronological age and corresponds to the 50th percentile in intellectual ability for the general population.

Intelligence tests assess cognitive function by evaluating comprehension, fund of knowledge, math skills, vocabulary, picture assembly, and other verbal and performance skills. Two common tests are:

Wechsler Adult Intelligence Scale (WAIS):
- Most common test for ages 16–90.
- Assesses overall intellectual functioning.
- Four index scores: Verbal comprehension, perceptual reasoning, working memory, processing speed.

Wechsler Intelligence Scale for Children (WISC): Tests intellectual ability in patients ages 6–16.

OBJECTIVE PERSONALITY ASSESSMENT TESTS

These tests are questions with standardized-answer format that can be objectively scored. The following is an example:

Minnesota Multiphasic Personality Inventory (MMPI-2)

- Tests personality for different pathologies and behavioral patterns.
- Most commonly used.

PROJECTIVE (PERSONALITY) ASSESSMENT TESTS

Projective tests have no structured-response format. The tests often ask for interpretation of ambiguous stimuli. Examples are:

Thematic Apperception Test (TAT)

- Test taker creates stories based on pictures of people in various situations.
- Used to evaluate motivations behind behaviors.

Rorschach Test

- Interpretation of inkblots.
- Used to identify thought disorders and defense mechanisms.

WARDS TIP

IQ Chart
Very superior: >130
Superior: 120–129
High average: 110–119
Average: 90–109
Low average: 80–89
Borderline: 70–79
Extremely low (intellectual disability): <70

CHAPTER 3

PSYCHOTIC DISORDERS

Psychosis	22
DELUSIONS	22
PERCEPTUAL DISTURBANCES	22
DIFFERENTIAL DIAGNOSIS OF PSYCHOSIS	22
PSYCHOTIC DISORDER DUE TO ANOTHER MEDICAL CONDITION	23
SUBSTANCE/MEDICATION-INDUCED PSYCHOTIC DISORDER	23
Schizophrenia	23
POSITIVE, NEGATIVE, AND COGNITIVE SYMPTOMS	24
THREE PHASES	24
DIAGNOSIS OF SCHIZOPHRENIA	24
PSYCHIATRIC EXAM OF PATIENTS WITH SCHIZOPHRENIA	25
EPIDEMIOLOGY	26
DOWNWARD DRIFT	26
PATHOPHYSIOLOGY OF SCHIZOPHRENIA: THE DOPAMINE HYPOTHESIS	26
OTHER NEUROTRANSMITTER ABNORMALITIES IMPLICATED IN SCHIZOPHRENIA	27
PROGNOSTIC FACTORS	27
TREATMENT	27
Schizophreniform Disorder	29
Schizoaffective Disorder	29
Brief Psychotic Disorder	30
Delusional Disorder	30
Culture-Specific Psychoses	31
Comparing Time Courses and Prognoses of Psychotic Disorders	31
QUICK AND EASY DISTINGUISHING FEATURES	31

Psychosis

Psychosis is a general term used to describe a distorted perception of reality. Poor reality testing may be accompanied by delusions, perceptual disturbances (illusions or hallucinations), and/or disorganized thinking/behavior. Psychosis can be a symptom of schizophrenia, mania, depression, delirium, and dementia, and it can be substance or medication-induced.

DELUSIONS

Delusions are fixed, false beliefs that remain despite evidence to the contrary and cannot be accounted for by the cultural background of the individual.

They can be categorized as either bizarre or nonbizarre. A *nonbizarre* delusion is a false belief that is plausible but is not true. Example: "The neighbors are spying on me by reading my mail." A *bizarre* delusion is a false belief that is impossible. Example: "A Martian fathered my baby and inserted a microchip in my brain."

Delusions can also be categorized by theme:

- **Delusions of persecution/paranoid delusions:** Irrational belief that one is being persecuted. Example: "The CIA is after me and tapped my phone."
- **Ideas of reference:** Belief that cues in the external environment are uniquely related to the individual. Example: "The TV characters are speaking directly to me."
- **Delusions of control:** Includes **thought broadcasting** (belief that one's thoughts can be heard by others) and **thought insertion** (belief that others' thoughts are being placed in one's head).
- **Delusions of grandeur:** Belief that one has special powers beyond those of a normal person. Example: "I am the all-powerful son of God and I shall bring down my wrath on you if I don't get my way."
- **Delusions of guilt:** Belief that one is guilty or responsible for something. Example: "I am responsible for all the world's wars."
- **Somatic delusions:** Belief that one is infected with a disease or has a certain illness.

PERCEPTUAL DISTURBANCES

- **Illusion:** Misinterpretation of an existing sensory stimulus (such as mistaking a shadow for a cat).
- **Hallucination:** Sensory perception without an actual external stimulus.
  - **Auditory:** Most commonly exhibited by schizophrenic patients.
  - **Visual:** Occurs but less common in schizophrenia. May accompany drug intoxication, drug and alcohol withdrawal, or delirium.
  - **Olfactory:** Usually an aura associated with epilepsy.
  - **Tactile:** Usually secondary to drug use or alcohol withdrawal.

DIFFERENTIAL DIAGNOSIS OF PSYCHOSIS

- Psychotic disorder due to another medical condition
- Substance/Medication-induced psychotic disorder
- Delirium/Dementia
- Bipolar disorder, manic/mixed episode
- Major depression with psychotic features

- Brief psychotic disorder
- Schizophrenia
- Schizophreniform disorder
- Schizoaffective disorder
- Delusional disorder

PSYCHOTIC DISORDER DUE TO ANOTHER MEDICAL CONDITION

Medical causes of psychosis include:

1. *Central nervous system (CNS) disease* (cerebrovascular disease, multiple sclerosis, neoplasm, Alzheimer's disease, Parkinson's disease, Huntington's disease, tertiary syphilis, epilepsy [often temporal lobe], encephalitis, prion disease, neurosarcoidosis, AIDS).
2. *Endocrinopathies* (Addison/Cushing disease, hyper/hypothyroidism, hyper/hypocalcemia, hypopituitarism).
3. *Nutritional/Vitamin deficiency states* (B12, folate, niacin).
4. *Other* (connective tissue disease [systemic lupus erythematosus, temporal arteritis], porphyria).

DSM-5 criteria for psychotic disorder due to another medical condition include:

- Prominent hallucinations or delusions.
- Symptoms do not occur only during an episode of delirium.
- Evidence from history, physical, or lab data to support another medical cause (i.e., not psychiatric).

SUBSTANCE/MEDICATION-INDUCED PSYCHOTIC DISORDER

Prescription medications that may cause psychosis in some patients include anesthetics, antimicrobials, corticosteroids, antiparkinsonian agents, anticonvulsants, antihistamines, anticholingerics, antihypertensives, NSAIDs, digitalis, methylphenidate, and chemotherapeutic agents. Substances such as alcohol, cocaine, hallucinogens (LSD, Ecstasy), cannabis, benzodiazepines, barbiturates, inhalants, and phencyclidine (PCP) can cause psychosis, either in intoxication or withdrawal.

DSM-5 Criteria

- Hallucinations and/or delusions.
- Symptoms do not occur only during episode of delirium.
- Evidence from history, physical, or lab data to support a medication or substance-induced cause.
- Disturbance is not better accounted for by a psychotic disorder that is not substance/medication-induced.

Schizophrenia

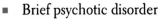 A 24-year-old male graduate student without prior medical or psychiatric history is reported by his mother to have been very anxious over the past 9 months, with increasing concern that people are watching him. He now claims to "hear voices" telling him what must be done to "fix the country." *Important workup?* Thyroid-stimulating hormone (TSH), rapid plasma reagin (RPR), brain imaging. *Likely diagnosis?* Schizophrenia. *Next step?* Antipsychotics.

WARDS TIP

It's important to be able to distinguish between a delusion, illusion, and hallucination. A delusion is a false belief, an illusion is a misinterpretation of an external stimulus, and a hallucination is perception in the absence of an external stimulus.

WARDS TIP

Elderly, medically ill patients who present with psychotic symptoms such as hallucinations, confusion, or paranoia should be carefully evaluated for delirium, which is a far more common finding in this population.

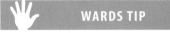
WARDS TIP

To make the diagnosis of schizophrenia, a patient must have symptoms of the disease for at least 6 months.

Schizophrenia is a psychiatric disorder characterized by a constellation of abnormalities in thinking, emotion, and behavior. There is no single symptom that is pathognomonic, and there is a heterogeneous clinical presentation. Schizophrenia is typically chronic, with significant psychosocial and medical consequences to the patient.

POSITIVE, NEGATIVE, AND COGNITIVE SYMPTOMS

In general, the symptoms of schizophrenia are broken up into three categories:

- **Positive symptoms:** Hallucinations, delusions, bizarre behavior, disorganized speech. These tend to respond more robustly to antipsychotic medications.
- **Negative symptoms:** Flat or blunted affect, anhedonia, apathy, alogia, and lack of interest in socialization. These symptoms are comparatively more often treatment resistant and contribute significantly to the social isolation of schizophrenic patients.
- **Cognitive symptoms:** Impairments in attention, executive function, and working memory. These symptoms may → poor work and school performance.

THREE PHASES

Symptoms of schizophrenia often present in three phases:

1. **Prodromal:** Decline in functioning that precedes the first psychotic episode. The patient may become socially withdrawn and irritable. He or she may have physical complaints, declining school/work performance, and/or newfound interest in religion or the occult.
2. **Psychotic:** Perceptual disturbances, delusions, and disordered thought process/content.
3. **Residual:** Occurs following an episode of active psychosis. It is marked by mild hallucinations or delusions, social withdrawal, and negative symptoms.

DIAGNOSIS OF SCHIZOPHRENIA

DSM-5 Criteria

- *Two or more* of the following must be present for at least *1 month:*
    1. Delusions
    2. Hallucinations
    3. Disorganized speech
    4. Grossly disorganized or catatonic behavior
    5. Negative symptoms
    Note: At least one must be **1, 2,** or **3.**
- Must cause significant social, occupational, or self-care functional deterioration.
- Duration of illness for at least 6 months (including prodromal or residual periods in which the above full criteria may not be met).
- Symptoms not due to effects of a substance or another medical condition.

 Mr. Torres is a 21-year-old man who is brought to the ER by his mother after he began talking about "aliens" who were trying to steal his soul. Mr. Torres reports that aliens left messages for him by arranging sticks outside his home and sometimes send thoughts into his mind.

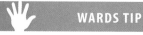

KEY FACT

Think of positive symptoms as things that are ADDED onto normal behavior. Think of negative symptoms as things that are SUBTRACTED or missing from normal behavior.

WARDS TIP

Stereotyped movement, bizarre posturing, and muscle rigidity are examples of catatonia seen in schizophrenic patients.

KEY FACT

Clozapine is typically considered for treating schizophrenia when a patient fails both typical and other atypical antipsychotics; this is due to the potential rare adverse event, agranulocytosis, which requires patients be monitored (WBC and ANC counts) regularly.

WARDS TIP

The 5 A's of schizophrenia (negative symptoms):
1. Anhedonia
2. Affect (flat)
3. Alogia (poverty of speech)
4. Avolition (apathy)
5. Attention (poor)

On exam, he is guarded and often stops talking while in the middle of expressing a thought. Mr. Torres appears anxious and frequently scans the room for aliens, which he thinks may have followed him to the hospital. He denies any plan to harm himself, but admits that the aliens sometimes want him to throw himself in front of a car, "as this will change the systems that belong under us."

The patient's mother reports that he began expressing these ideas a few months ago, but that they have become more severe in the last few weeks. She reports that during the past year, he has become isolated from his peers, frequently talks to himself, and has stopped going to community college. He has also spent most of his time reading science fiction books and creating devices that will prevent aliens from hurting him. She reports that she is concerned because the patient's father, who left while the patient was a child, exhibited similar symptoms many years ago and has spent most of his life in psychiatric hospitals.

What is Mr. Torres's most likely diagnosis? What differential diagnoses should be considered?

Mr. Torres's most likely diagnosis is schizophrenia. He exhibits delusional ideas that are bizarre and paranoid in nature. He also reports the presence of frequent auditory hallucinations and disturbances in thought process that include thought blocking. Although the patient's mother reports that his psychotic symptoms began "a few months ago," the patient has exhibited social and occupational dysfunction during the last year. Mr. Torres quit school, became isolated, and has been responding to internal stimuli since that time. In addition, his father appears to also suffer from a psychotic disorder. In this case, it appears that the disorder has been present for more than 6 months; however, if this is unclear, the diagnosis of schizophreniform disorder should be made instead.

The differential diagnosis should also include schizoaffective disorder, medication/substance-induced psychotic disorder, psychotic disorder due to another medical condition, and mood disorder with psychotic features.

What would be appropriate steps in the acute management of this patient?

Treatment should include inpatient hospitalization in order to provide a safe environment, with monitoring of suicidal ideation secondary to his psychosis. Routine laboratory tests, including a urine or serum drug screen, should be undertaken. The patient should begin treatment with antipsychotic medication while closely being monitored for potential side effects.

PSYCHIATRIC EXAM OF PATIENTS WITH SCHIZOPHRENIA

The typical findings in schizophrenic patients include:

- Disheveled appearance
- Flat affect
- Disorganized thought process

WARDS TIP

Echolalia—repeats words or phrases
EchoPRAxia—mimics behavior
(PRActices behavior)

KEY FACT

Brief psychotic disorder lasts for < 1 month. Schizophreniform disorder can last between 1 and 6 months. Schizophrenia lasts for > 6 months.

- Intact procedural memory and orientation
- Auditory hallucinations
- Paranoid delusions
- Ideas of reference
- Lack of insight into their disease

EPIDEMIOLOGY

- Schizophrenia affects approximately 0.3–0.7% of people over their lifetime.
- Men and women are equally affected but have different presentations and outcomes:
  - Men tend to present in early to mid-20s
  - Women present in late 20s
  - Men tend to have more negative symptoms and poorer outcome compared to women.
- Schizophrenia rarely presents before age 15 or after age 55.
- There is a strong genetic predisposition:
  - 50% concordance rate among monozygotic twins
  - 40% risk of inheritance if both parents have schizophrenia
  - 12% risk if one first-degree relative is affected
- Substance use is comorbid in many patients with schizophrenia. The most commonly abused substance is nicotine (>50%), followed by alcohol, cannabis, and cocaine.
- Post-psychotic depression is the phenomenon of schizophrenic patients developing a major depressive episode after resolution of their psychotic symptoms.

DOWNWARD DRIFT

Lower socioeconomic groups have higher rates of schizophrenia. This may be due to the **downward drift hypothesis**, which postulates that people suffering from schizophrenia are unable to function well in society and hence end up in lower socioeconomic groups. Many homeless people in urban areas suffer from schizophrenia.

PATHOPHYSIOLOGY OF SCHIZOPHRENIA: THE DOPAMINE HYPOTHESIS

Though the exact cause of schizophrenia is not known, it appears to be partly related to ↑ dopamine activity in certain neuronal tracts. Evidence to support this hypothesis is that most antipsychotics successful in treating schizophrenia are dopamine receptor antagonists. In addition, cocaine and amphetamines ↑ dopamine activity and can → schizophrenic-like symptoms.

Theorized Dopamine Pathways Affected in Schizophrenia

- *Prefrontal cortical:* Inadequate dopaminergic activity responsible for negative symptoms.
- *Mesolimbic:* Excessive dopaminergic activity responsible for positive symptoms.

Other Important Dopamine Pathways Affected by antipsychotics

- *Tuberoinfundibular:* Blocked by antipsychotics, causing hyperprolactinemia, which may → gynecomastia, galactorrhea, sexual dysfunction, and menstrual irregularities.
- *Nigrostriatal:* Blocked by antipsychotics, causing Parkinsonism/extrapyramidal side effects such as tremor, rigidity, slurred speech, akathisia, dystonia, and other abnormal movements.

OTHER NEUROTRANSMITTER ABNORMALITIES IMPLICATED IN SCHIZOPHRENIA

- **Elevated serotonin:** Some of the second-generation (atypical) antipsychotics (e.g., risperidone and clozapine) antagonize serotonin and weakly antagonize dopamine.
- **Elevated norepinephrine:** Long-term use of antipsychotics has been shown to ↓ activity of noradrenergic neurons.
- **↓ gamma-aminobutyric acid (GABA):** There is ↓ expression of the enzyme necessary to create GABA in the hippocampus of schizophrenic patients.
- **↓ levels of glutamate receptors:** Schizophrenic patients have fewer NMDA receptors; this corresponds to the psychotic symptoms observed with NMDA antagonists like ketamine.

PROGNOSTIC FACTORS

Even with medication, 40–60% of patients remain significantly impaired after their diagnosis, while only 20–30% function fairly well in society. About 20% of patients with schizophrenia attempt suicide and many more experience suicidal ideation. Several factors are associated with a better or worse prognosis:

Associated with Better Prognosis
- Later onset
- Good social support
- Positive symptoms
- Mood symptoms
- Acute onset
- Female gender
- Few relapses
- Good premorbid functioning

Associated with Worse Prognosis
- Early onset
- Poor social support
- Negative symptoms
- Family history
- Gradual onset
- Male gender
- Many relapses
- Poor premorbid functioning (social isolation, etc.)
- Comorbid substance use

TREATMENT

A multimodal approach is the most effective, and therapy must be tailored to the needs of the specific patient. **Pharmacologic** treatment consists primarily of antipsychotic medications, otherwise known as neuroleptics. (For more detail, see the Psychopharmacology chapter.)

- **First-generation (or typical) antipsychotic medications** (e.g., *chlorpromazine, fluphenazine, haloperidol, perphenazine*):
    - These are primarily dopamine (mostly D2) antagonists.
    - Treat positive symptoms with minimal impact on negative symptoms.
    - Side effects include extrapyramidal symptoms, neuroleptic malignant syndrome, and tardive dyskinesia (see below).

KEY FACT

Schizophrenia has a large genetic component. If one identical twin has schizophrenia, the risk of the other identical twin having schizophrenia is 50%. A biological child of a schizophrenic person has a higher chance of developing schizophrenia, even if adopted.

KEY FACT

Computed tomographic (CT) and magnetic resonance imaging (MRI) scans of patients with schizophrenia may show enlargement of the ventricles and diffuse cortical atrophy and reduced brain volume.

KEY FACT

Schizophrenia often involves neologisms. A neologism is a newly coined word or expression that has meaning only to the person who uses it.

WARDS TIP

First-generation antipsychotic medications are referred to as typical or conventional antipsychotics (often called neuroleptics). Second-generation antipsychotic medications are referred to as atypical antipsychotics.

Schizophrenic patients who are treated with *second-generation* (atypical) antipsychotic medications need a careful medical evaluation for metabolic syndrome. This includes checking weight, body mass index (BMI), fasting blood glucose, lipid assessment, and blood pressure.

WARDS TIP

Patients who are treated with *first-generation* (typical) antipsychotic medication need to be closely monitored for extrapyramidal symptoms, such as acute dystonia and tardive dyskinesia.

KEY FACT

High-potency antipsychotics (such as haloperidol and fluphenazine) have a higher incidence of extrapyramidal side effects, while *low-potency* antipsychotics (such as chlorpromazine) have primarily anticholinergic and antiadrenergic side effects.

WARDS TIP

Tardive dyskinesia occurs most often in older women after at least 6 months of medication. A small percentage of patients will experience spontaneous remission, so discontinuation of the agent should be considered if clinically appropriate.

- **Second-generation (or atypical) antipsychotic medications** (e.g., *aripiprazole, asenapine, clozapine, iloperidone, lurasidone, olanzapine, quetiapine, risperidone, ziprasidone*):
  - These antagonize serotonin receptors (5-HT2) as well as dopamine (D4>D2) receptors.
  - Research has shown no significant difference between first- and second-generation antipsychotics in efficacy. The selection requires the weighing of benefits and risks in individual clinical cases.
  - Lower incidence of extrapyramidal side effects, but ↑ risk for metabolic syndrome.
  - Medications should be taken for at least 4 weeks before efficacy is determined.
  - Clozapine is reserved for patients who have failed multiple antipsychotic trials due to its ↑ risk of agranulocytosis.

Behavioral therapy attempts to improve patients' ability to function in society. Patients are helped through a variety of methods to improve their social skills, become self-sufficient, and minimize disruptive behaviors. **Family therapy** and **group therapy** are also useful adjuncts.

Important Side Effects and Sequelae of Antipsychotic Medications

Side effects of antipsychotic medications include:

1. Extrapyramidal symptoms (especially with the use of high-potency first-generation antipsychotics):
   - Dystonia (spasms) of face, neck, and tongue
   - Parkinsonism (resting tremor, rigidity, bradykinesia)
   - Akathisia (feeling of restlessness)
   Treatment: Anticholinergics (benztropine, diphenhydramine), benzodiazepines/beta-blockers (specifically for akathisia)
2. Anticholinergic symptoms (especially low-potency first-generation antipsychotics and atypical antipsychotics): Dry mouth, constipation, blurred vision, hyperthermia.
   Treatment: As per symptom (eye drops, stool softeners, etc.)
3. Metabolic syndrome (second-generation antipsychotics): A constellation of conditions—↑ blood pressure, ↑ blood sugar levels, excess body fat around the waist, abnormal cholesterol levels—that occur together, ↑ the risk for developing cardiovascular disease, stroke, and type 2 diabetes.
   Treatment: Consider switching to a first-generation antipsychotic or a more "weight-neutral" second-generation antipsychotic such as aripiprazole or ziprasidone. Monitor lipids and blood glucose measurements. Refer the patient to primary care for appropriate treatment of hyperlipidemia, diabetes, etc. Encourage appropriate diet, exercise, and smoking cessation.
4. Tardive dyskinesia (more likely with first-generation antipsychotics): Choreoathetoid movements, usually seen in the face, tongue, and head.
   Treatment: Discontinue or reduce the medication and consider substituting an atypical antipsychotic (if appropriate). Benzodiazepines, Botox, and vitamin E may be used. The movements may persist despite withdrawal of the drug. Although less common, atypical antipsychotics can cause tardive dyskinesia.
5. Neuroleptic malignant syndrome (typically high-potency first-generation antipsychotics):
   - Change in mental status, autonomic instability (high fever, labile blood pressure, tachycardia, tachypnea, diaphoresis), "lead pipe" rigidity, elevated creatine phosphokinase (CPK) levels, leukocytosis, and metabolic acidosis.
   - A medical emergency that requires prompt withdrawal of all antipsychotic medications and immediate medical assessment and treatment.
   - May be observed in any patient being treated with any antipsychotic (including second generation) medications at any time, but is more

frequently associated with the initiation of treatment and at higher IV/
IM dosing of high-potency neuroleptics.

- Patients with a history of prior neuroleptic malignant syndrome are at
  an ↑ risk of recurrent episodes when retrialed with antipsychotic agents.

6. Prolonged QTc interval and other electrocardiogram changes, hyperprolactinemia (→ gynecomastia, galactorrhea, amenorrhea, diminished
libido, and impotence), hematologic effects (agranulocytosis may occur
with *clozapine*, requiring frequent blood draws when this medication
is used), ophthalmologic conditions (*thioridazine* may cause irreversible retinal pigmentation at high doses; deposits in lens and cornea may
occur with *chlorpromazine*), dermatologic conditions (such as rashes and
photosensitivity).

Schizophreniform Disorder

Diagnosis and DSM-5 Criteria

The diagnosis of schizophreniform disorder is made using the same DSM-5
criteria as schizophrenia. The only difference between the two is that in
schizophreniform disorder the symptoms have lasted between 1 and 6 months,
whereas in schizophrenia the symptoms must be present for > 6 months.

Prognosis

One-third of patients recover completely; two-thirds progress to schizoaffective disorder or schizophrenia.

Treatment

Hospitalization (if necessary), 6-month course of antipsychotics, and supportive psychotherapy.

Schizoaffective Disorder

Diagnosis and DSM-5 Criteria

The diagnosis of schizoaffective disorder is made in patients who:
- Meet criteria for either a major depressive or manic episode during which
  psychotic symptoms consistent with schizophrenia are also met.
- Delusions or hallucinations for 2 weeks in the absence of mood disorder
  symptoms (this criterion is necessary to differentiate schizoaffective disorder from mood disorder with psychotic features).
- Mood symptoms present for a majority of the psychotic illness.
- Symptoms not due to the effects of a substance (drug or medication) or
  another medical condition.

Prognosis

Worse with poor premorbid adjustment, slow onset, early onset, predominance
of psychotic symptoms, long course, and family history of schizophrenia.

Treatment

- Hospitalization (if necessary) and supportive psychotherapy.
- Medical therapy: Antipsychotics (second-generation medications may
  target both psychotic and mood symptoms); mood stabilizers, antidepressants, or electroconvulsive therapy (ECT) may be indicated for treatment
  of mood symptoms.

Brief Psychotic Disorder

Diagnosis and DSM-5 Criteria

Patient with psychotic symptoms as in schizophrenia; however, the symptoms last from 1 day to 1 month, and there must be eventual full return to premorbid level of functioning. Symptoms must not be due to the effects of a substance (drug or medication) or another medical condition. This is a rare diagnosis, much less common than schizophrenia. It may be seen in reaction to extreme stress such as bereavement, sexual assault, etc.

Prognosis

High rates of relapse, but almost all completely recover.

Treatment

Brief hospitalization (usually required for workup, safety, and stabilization), supportive therapy, course of antipsychotics for psychosis, and/or benzodiazepines for agitation.

Delusional Disorder

Delusional disorder occurs more often in middle-aged or older patients (after age 40). Immigrants, the hearing impaired, and those with a family history of schizophrenia are at increased risk.

Diagnosis and DSM-5 Criteria

To be diagnosed with delusional disorder, the following criteria must be met:

- One or more delusions for at least 1 month.
- Does not meet criteria for schizophrenia.
- Functioning in life not significantly impaired, and behavior not obviously bizarre.
- While delusions may be present in both delusional disorder and schizophrenia, there are important differences (see Table 3-1).

Types of Delusions

Patients are further categorized based on the types of delusions they experience:

- **Erotomanic type:** Delusion that another person is in love with the individual.
- **Grandiose type:** Delusions of having great talent.
- **Somatic type:** Physical delusions.
- **Persecutory type:** Delusions of being persecuted.

TABLE 3-1. **Schizophrenia versus Delusional Disorder**

SCHIZOPHRENIA	DELUSIONAL DISORDER
■ Bizarre or nonbizarre delusions	■ Usually nonbizarre delusions
■ Daily functioning significantly impaired	■ Daily functioning not significantly impaired
■ Must have two or more of the following:	■ Does not meet the criteria for schizophrenia as described in the left column
■ Delusions	
■ Hallucinations	
■ Disorganized speech	
■ Disorganized behavior	
■ Negative symptoms	

- **Jealous type:** Delusions of unfaithfulness.
- **Mixed type:** More than one of the above.
- **Unspecified type:** Not a specific type as described above.

Prognosis

- Better than schizophrenia with treatment:
- > 50%: Full recovery
- > 20%: ↓ symptoms
- < 20%: No change

Treatment

Difficult to treat, especially given the lack of insight and impairment. Antipsychotic medications are recommended despite somewhat limited evidence. Supportive therapy is often helpful, but group therapy should be avoided given the patient's suspiciousness.

Culture-Specific Psychoses

The following are examples of psychotic disorders seen within certain cultures:

	PSYCHOTIC MANIFESTATION	CULTURE
Koro	Intense anxiety that the penis will recede into the body, possibly leading to death.	Southeast Asia (e.g., Singapore)
Amok	Sudden unprovoked outbursts of violence, often followed by suicide.	Malaysia
Brain fag	Headache, fatigue, eye pain, cognitive difficulties, and other somatic disturbances in male students.	Africa

Comparing Time Courses and Prognoses of Psychotic Disorders

Time Course

- < 1 month—brief psychotic disorder
- 1–6 months—schizophreniform disorder
- > 6 months—schizophrenia

Prognosis from Best to Worst

Mood disorder with psychotic features > schizoaffective disorder > schizophreniform disorder > schizophrenia.

QUICK AND EASY DISTINGUISHING FEATURES

- **Schizophrenia:** Lifelong psychotic disorder.
- **Schizophreniform:** Schizophrenia for > 1 and < 6 months.
- **Schizoaffective:** Schizophrenia + mood disorder.
- **Schizotypal** (personality disorder): Paranoid, odd or magical beliefs, eccentric, lack of friends, social anxiety. Criteria for overt psychosis are not met.
- **Schizoid** (personality disorder): Solitary activities, lack of enjoyment from social interactions, no psychosis.

KEY FACT

SchizophreniFORM = the FORMation of a schizophrenic, but not quite there (i.e., < 6 months).

NOTES

CHAPTER 4

MOOD DISORDERS

Concepts in Mood Disorders	34
Mood Disorders versus Mood Episodes	34
Mood Episodes	34
MAJOR DEPRESSIVE EPISODE (DSM-5 CRITERIA)	34
MANIC EPISODE (DSM-5 CRITERIA)	34
HYPOMANIC EPISODE	35
DIFFERENCES BETWEEN MANIC AND HYPOMANIC EPISODES	35
MIXED FEATURES	35
Mood Disorders	35
DIFFERENTIAL DIAGNOSIS OF MOOD DISORDERS DUE TO OTHER MEDICAL CONDITIONS	35
SUBSTANCE/MEDICATION-INDUCED MOOD DISORDERS	36
MAJOR DEPRESSIVE DISORDER (MDD)	36
SPECIFIERS FOR DEPRESSIVE DISORDERS	39
BEREAVEMENT	40
BIPOLAR I DISORDER	40
BIPOLAR II DISORDER	41
SPECIFIERS FOR BIPOLAR DISORDERS	42
PERSISTENT DEPRESSIVE DISORDER (DYSTHYMIA)	42
CYCLOTHYMIC DISORDER	43
PREMENSTRUAL DYSPHORIC DISORDER	43
DISRUPTIVE MOOD DYSREGULATION DISORDER (DMDD)	44
OTHER DISORDERS OF MOOD IN DSM-5	45

Concepts in Mood Disorders

A **mood** is a description of one's internal emotional state. Both external and internal stimuli can trigger moods, which may be labeled as sad, happy, angry, irritable, and so on. It is normal to have a wide range of moods and to have a sense of control over one's moods.

Patients with mood *disorders* (also called affective disorders) experience an abnormal range of moods and lose some level of control over them. Distress may be caused by the severity of their moods and the resulting impairment in social and occupational functioning.

Mood Disorders versus Mood Episodes

- **Mood episodes** are distinct periods of time in which some abnormal mood is present. They include depression, mania, and hypomania.
- **Mood disorders** are defined by their patterns of mood episodes. They include major depressive disorder (MDD), bipolar I disorder, bipolar II disorder, persistent depressive disorder, and cyclothymic disorder. Some may have psychotic features (delusions or hallucinations).

Mood Episodes

MAJOR DEPRESSIVE EPISODE (DSM-5 CRITERIA)

Must have at least five of the following symptoms (must include either number 1 or 2) for at least a 2-week period:

1. Depressed mood most of the time
2. Anhedonia (loss of interest in pleasurable activities)
3. Change in appetite or weight ($\uparrow$ or $\downarrow$)
4. Feelings of worthlessness or excessive guilt
5. Insomnia or hypersomnia
6. Diminished concentration
7. Psychomotor agitation or retardation (i.e., restlessness or slowness)
8. Fatigue or loss of energy
9. Recurrent thoughts of death or suicide

Symptoms are not attributable to the effects of a substance (drug or medication) or another medical condition, and they must cause clinically significant distress or social/occupational impairment.

MANIC EPISODE (DSM-5 CRITERIA)

A distinct period of abnormally and persistently elevated, expansive, or irritable mood, and abnormally and persistently increased goal-directed activity or energy, lasting at least 1 week (or any duration if hospitalization is necessary), and including at least three of the following (four if mood is only irritable):

1. Distractibility
2. Inflated self-esteem or grandiosity
3. $\uparrow$ in goal-directed activity (socially, at work, or sexually) or psychomotor agitation

4. ↓ need for sleep
5. Flight of ideas or racing thoughts
6. More talkative than usual or *pressured speech* (rapid and uninterruptible)
7. Excessive involvement in pleasurable activities that have a high risk of negative consequences (e.g., shopping sprees, sexual indiscretions)

Symptoms are not attributable to the effects of a substance (drug or medication) or another medical condition, and they must cause clinically significant distress or social/occupational impairment. Greater than 50% of manic patients have psychotic symptoms.

HYPOMANIC EPISODE

A hypomanic episode is a distinct period of abnormally and persistently elevated, expansive, or irritable mood, and abnormally and persistently increased goal-directed activity or energy, lasting at least 4 consecutive days, that includes at least three of the symptoms listed for the manic episode criteria (four if mood is only irritable). There are significant differences between mania and hypomania (see below).

DIFFERENCES BETWEEN MANIC AND HYPOMANIC EPISODES

Mania	Hypomania
Lasts at least 7 days	Lasts at least 4 days
Causes severe impairment in social or occupational functioning	No marked impairment in social or occupational functioning
May necessitate hospitalization to prevent harm to self or others	Does not require hospitalization
May have psychotic features	No psychotic features

MIXED FEATURES

Criteria are met for a manic or hypomanic episode and at least three symptoms of a major depressive episode are present for the majority of the time. These criteria must be present nearly every day for at least 1 week.

Mood Disorders

Mood disorders often have chronic courses that are marked by relapses *with relatively normal functioning between episodes*. Like most psychiatric diagnoses, mood episodes may be caused by another medical condition or drug (prescribed or illicit); therefore, always investigate medical or substance-induced causes (see below) before making a primary psychiatric diagnosis.

DIFFERENTIAL DIAGNOSIS OF MOOD DISORDERS DUE TO OTHER MEDICAL CONDITIONS

Medical Causes of a Depressive Episode	Medical Causes of a Manic Episode
Cerebrovascular disease (stroke, myocardial infarction)	Metabolic (hyperthyroidism)
Endocrinopathies (diabetes mellitus, Cushing syndrome, Addison disease,	Neurological disorders (temporal lobe seizures, multiple sclerosis)

hypoglycemia,
hyper/hypothyroidism,
hyper/hypocalcemia)
Parkinson's disease
Viral illnesses (e.g., mononucleosis)
Carcinoid syndrome
Cancer (especially lymphoma and
pancreatic carcinoma)
Collagen vascular disease (e.g.,
systemic lupus erythematosus)

Neoplasms
HIV infection

SUBSTANCE/MEDICATION-INDUCED MOOD DISORDERS

Substance/Medication-Induced Depressive Disorder

EtOH
Antihypertensives
Barbiturates
Corticosteroids
Levodopa
Sedative-hypnotics
Anticonvulsants
Antipsychotics
Diuretics
Sulfonamides
Withdrawal from
    stimulants (e.g., cocaine,
    amphetamines)

Substance/Medication-Induced Bipolar Disorder

Antidepressants
Sympathomimetics
Dopamine
Corticosteroids
Levodopa
Bronchodilators
Cocaine
Amphetamines

MAJOR DEPRESSIVE DISORDER (MDD)

MDD is marked by episodes of depressed mood associated with loss of interest in daily activities. Patients may not acknowledge their depressed mood or may express vague, somatic complaints (fatigue, headache, abdominal pain, muscle tension, etc.).

Diagnosis and DSM-5 Criteria

- At least one major depressive episode (see above).
- No history of manic or hypomanic episode.

Epidemiology

- Lifetime prevalence: 12% worldwide.
- Onset at any age, but the age of onset peaks in the 20s.
- 1.5–2 times as prevalent in women than men during reproductive years.
- No ethnic or socioeconomic differences.
- Lifetime prevalence in the elderly: <10%.
- Depression can ↑ mortality for patients with other comorbidities such as diabetes, stroke, and cardiovascular disease.

Sleep Problems Associated with MDD

- Multiple awakenings.
- Initial and terminal insomnia (hard to fall asleep and early morning awakenings).
- Hypersomnia (excessive sleepiness) is less common.
- Rapid eye movement (REM) sleep shifted earlier in the night and for a greater duration, with reduced stages 3 and 4 (slow wave) sleep.

KEY FACT

Stroke patients are at a significant risk for developing depression, and this is associated with a poorer outcome overall.

KEY FACT

Major depressive disorder is the most common disorder among those who complete suicide.

KEY FACT

Most adults with depression do not see a mental health professional, but they often present to a primary care physician for other reasons.

KEY FACT

Anhedonia is the inability to experience pleasure, which is a common finding in depression.

Etiology

The precise cause of depression is unknown, but MDD is believed to be a heterogeneous disease, with biological, genetic, environmental, and psychosocial factors contributing.

- MDD is likely caused by neurotransmitter abnormalities in the brain. Evidence for this is the following: antidepressants exert their therapeutic effect by increasing catecholamines; ↓ cerebrospinal fluid (CSF) levels of 5-hydroxyindolacetic acid (5-HIAA), the main metabolite of serotonin, have been found in depressed patients with impulsive and suicidal behavior.
- Increased sensitivity of beta-adrenergic receptors in the brain has also been postulated in the pathogenesis of MDD.
- **High cortisol:** Hyperactivity of hypothalamic-pituitary-adrenal axis, as shown by failure to suppress cortisol levels in the dexamethasone suppression test.
- **Abnormal thyroid axis:** Thyroid disorders are associated with depressive symptoms.
- Gamma-aminobutyric acid (GABA), glutamate, and endogenous opiates may additionally have a role.
- **Psychosocial/life events:** Multiple adverse childhood experiences are a risk factor for later developing MDD.
- **Genetics:** First-degree relatives are two to four times more likely to have MDD. Concordance rate for monozygotic twins is <40%, and 10–20% for dizygotic twins.

Course and Prognosis

- Untreated, depressive episodes are self-limiting but last from 6 to 12 months. Generally, episodes occur more frequently as the disorder progresses. The risk of a subsequent major depressive episode is 50–60% within the first 2 years after the first episode. 2–12% of patients with MDD eventually commit suicide.
- Approximately 60% of patients show a significant response to antidepressants. Combined treatment with both an antidepressant and psychotherapy produce a significantly ↑ response for MDD.

Treatment

Hospitalization

- Indicated if patient is at risk for suicide, homicide, or is unable to care for him/herself.

Pharmacotherapy

- **Antidepressant medications:**
  - *Selective serotonin reuptake inhibitors (SSRIs):* Safer and better tolerated than other classes of antidepressants; side effects are mild but include headache, *gastrointestinal disturbance*, *sexual dysfunction*, and rebound anxiety. Medications that also have activation of other neurotransmitters include serotonin-norepinephrine reuptake inhibitors venlafaxine (Effexor) and duloxetine (Cymbalta), the α2-adrenergic receptor antagonist mirtazapine (Remeron), and the dopamine-norepinephrine reuptake inhibitor bupropion (Wellbutrin).
  - *Tricyclic antidepressants (TCAs):* Most lethal in overdose due to cardiac arrhythmias; side effects include sedation, weight gain, orthostatic hypotension, and anticholinergic effects. Can aggravate prolonged QTc syndrome.
  - *Monoamine oxidase inhibitors (MAOIs):* Older medications occasionally used for refractory depression; risk of *hypertensive crisis* when used with sympathomimetics or ingestion of tyramine-rich foods, such as wine, beer, aged cheeses, liver, and smoked meats (tyramine is an intermediate in the conversion of tyrosine to norepinephrine); risk of

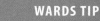

WARDS TIP

The two most common types of sleep disturbances associated with MDD are difficulty falling asleep and early morning awakenings.

KEY FACT

The Hamilton Depression Rating Scale measures the severity of depression and is used in research to assess the effectiveness of therapies. PHQ-9 is a depression screening form often used in the primary care setting.

KEY FACT

Loss of a parent before age 11 is associated with the later development of major depression.

KEY FACT

Depression is common in patients with pancreatic cancer.

KEY FACT

Only half of patients with MDD receive treatment.

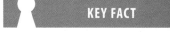
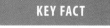

KEY FACT

All antidepressant medications are equally effective but differ in side-effect profiles. Medications usually take 4–6 weeks to fully work.

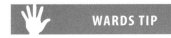

WARDS TIP

Serotonin syndrome is marked by autonomic instability, hyperthermia, hyperreflexia (including myoclonus), and seizures. Coma or death may result.

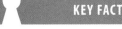

WARDS TIP

Adjunctive treatment is usually performed after multiple first-line treatment failures.

KEY FACT

Postpartum period conveys an elevated risk of depression in women.

WARDS TIP

MAOIs were considered particularly useful in the treatment of "atypical" depression; however, SSRIs remain first-line treatment for major depressive episodes with atypical features.

serotonin syndrome when used in combination with SSRIs. Most common side effect is orthostatic hypotension.

- **Adjunct medications:**
  - Atypical (second-generation) antipsychotics along with antidepressants are first-line treatment in patients with MDD with psychotic features. In addition, they may also be prescribed in patients with treatment resistant/refractory MDD without psychotic features.
  - Triiodothyronine (T_3), levothyroxine (T_4), and lithium have demonstrated some benefit when augmenting antidepressants in treatment refractory MDD.
  - While stimulants (such as methylphenidate) may be used in certain patients (e.g., terminally ill), the efficacy is limited and trials are small.

Psychotherapy
- Cognitive-behavioral therapy (CBT), interpersonal psychotherapy, supportive therapy, psychodynamic psychotherapy, problem-solving therapy, and family/couples therapy have all demonstrated some benefit in treating MDD (primarily CBT or interpersonal psychotherapy).
- May be used alone or in conjunction with pharmacotherapy.

Electroconvulsive Therapy (ECT)
- Indicated if patient is unresponsive to pharmacotherapy, if patient cannot tolerate pharmacotherapy (pregnancy, etc.), or if rapid reduction of symptoms is desired (e.g., immediate suicide risk, refusal to eat/drink, catatonia).
- ECT is extremely safe (primary risk is from anesthesia) and may be used alone or in combination with pharmacotherapy.
- ECT is often performed by premedication with atropine, followed by general anesthesia (usually with methohexital) and administration of a muscle relaxant (typically succinylcholine). A generalized seizure is then induced by passing a current of electricity across the brain (generally bilateral, less commonly unilateral); the seizure should last between 30 and 60 seconds, and no longer than 90 seconds.
- 6–12 (average of 7) treatments are administered over a 2- to 3-week period, but significant improvement is sometimes noted after the first treatment.
- Retrograde and anterograde amnesia are common side effects, which usually resolve within 6 months.
- Other common but transient side effects: Headache, nausea, muscle soreness.

Ms. Cruz is a 28-year-old sales clerk who arrives at your outpatient clinic complaining of sadness after her boyfriend of 6 months ended their relationship 1 month ago. She describes a history of failed romantic relationships, and says, "I don't do well with breakups." Ms. Cruz reports that, although she has no prior psychiatric treatment, she was urged by her employer to seek therapy. Ms. Cruz has arrived late to work on several occasions because of oversleeping. She also has difficulty in getting out of bed stating, "It's difficult to walk; it's like my legs weigh a ton." She feels fatigued during the day despite spending over 12 hours in bed, and is concerned that she might be suffering from a serious medical condition. She denies any significant changes in appetite or weight since these symptoms began.

Ms. Cruz reports that, although she has not missed workdays, she has difficulty concentrating and has become tearful in front of clients while worrying about not finding a significant other. She feels tremendous guilt over "not being good enough to get married," and says that her close friends are concerned because she has been spending her weekends in bed and not answering their calls. Although during your evaluation Ms. Cruz appeared tearful, she brightened up when talking about her newborn nephew and her plans of visiting a college friend next summer. Ms. Cruz denied suicidal ideation.

What is Ms. Cruz's diagnosis?

Ms. Cruz's diagnosis is major depressive disorder with atypical features. She complains of sadness, fatigue, poor concentration, hypersomnia, feelings of guilt, anhedonia, and impairment in her social and occupational functioning. The atypical features specifier is given in this case as she exhibited mood reactivity (mood brightens in response to positive events) when talking about her nephew and visiting her friend, and complained of a heavy feeling in her legs (leaden paralysis) and hypersomnia. It is also important to explore Ms. Cruz's history of "not doing well with breakups," as this could be indicative of a long pattern of interpersonal rejection sensitivity. Although it is common for patients who suffer from atypical depression to report an ↑ in appetite, Ms. Cruz exhibits enough symptoms to fulfill atypical features criteria. Adjustment disorder should also be considered in the differential diagnosis.

What would be your pharmacological recommendation?

Ms. Cruz should be treated with an antidepressant medication. While MAOIs such as phenelzine had traditionally been superior to TCAs in the treatment of MDD with atypical features, SSRIs would be the first-line treatment. The combination of pharmacotherapy and psychotherapy has been shown to be more effective for treating mild-to-moderate MDD than either treatment alone.

SPECIFIERS FOR DEPRESSIVE DISORDERS

- **Melancholic features:** Present in approximately 25–30% of patients with MDE and more likely in severely ill inpatients, including those with psychotic features. Characterized by *anhedonia*, early morning awakenings, depression worse in the morning, psychomotor disturbance, excessive guilt, and anorexia. For example, you may diagnose major depressive disorder with melancholic features.
- **Atypical features:** Characterized by hypersomnia, hyperphagia, reactive mood, leaden paralysis, and hypersensitivity to interpersonal rejection.
- **Mixed features:** Manic/hypomanic symptoms present during the majority of days during MDE: elevated mood, grandiosity, talkativeness/pressured speech, flight of ideas/racing thoughts, increased energy/goal-directed activity, excessive involvement in dangerous activities, and decreased need for sleep.
- **Catatonia:** Features include catalepsy (immobility), purposeless motor activity, extreme negativism or mutism, bizarre postures, and echolalia. Especially responsive to ECT. (May also be applied to bipolar disorder.)
- **Psychotic features:** Characterized by the presence of delusions and/or hallucinations. Present in 24–53% of older, hospitalized patients with MDD.

Triad for seasonal affective disorder:
- Irritability
- Carbohydrate craving
- Hypersomnia

WARDS TIP

Major depression with psychotic features is best treated with a combination of antidepressant and antipsychotic or ECT

KEY FACT

Bereavement is NOT a DSM-5 diagnosis—if a patient meets criteria for major depression following the loss of a loved one, the diagnosis is major depression.

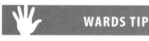

WARDS TIP

Bipolar I disorder may have psychotic features (delusions or hallucinations); these can occur during major depressive *or* manic episodes. Remember to always include bipolar disorder in the differential diagnoses of a psychotic patient.

KEY FACT

Rapid cycling is defined by the occurrence of four or more mood episodes in 1 year (major depressive, hypomanic, or manic).

- **Anxious distress:** Defined by feeling keyed up/tense, restless, difficulty concentrating, fears of something bad happening, and feelings of loss of control.
- **Peripartum onset:** Onset of MDD symptoms occurs during pregnancy or 4 weeks following delivery.
- **Seasonal pattern:** Temporal relationship between onset of MDD and particular time of the year (most commonly the winter but may occur in any season). Patients with fall-onset SAD (Seasonal affective disorder or "winter depression") often respond to light therapy.

BEREAVEMENT

Bereavement, also known as simple grief, is a reaction to a major loss, usually of a loved one, and it is not a mental illness. While symptoms are usually self-limited and only last for several months, if an individual meets criteria for a depressive episode, he/she would be diagnosed with MDD. Normal bereavement should not include gross psychotic symptoms, disorganization, or active suicidality.

BIPOLAR I DISORDER

Bipolar I disorder involves episodes of mania and of major depression; however, episodes of major depression are *not* required for the diagnosis. It is also known as **manic-depression**.

Diagnosis and DSM-5 Criteria

The only requirement for this diagnosis is the occurrence of a **manic episode** (5% of patients experience only manic episodes). Between manic episodes, there may be interspersed euthymia, major depressive episodes, or hypomanic episodes, but none of these are required for the diagnosis.

Epidemiology

- Lifetime prevalence: 1–2%.
- Women and men are equally affected.
- No ethnic differences seen; however, high-income countries have twice the rate of low-income countries (1.4% versus 0.7%).
- Onset usually before age 30, mean age of first mood episode is 18.
- Frequently misdiagnosed and thereby inappropriately or inadequately treated.

Etiology

- Biological, environmental, psychosocial, and genetic factors are all important.
- First-degree relatives of patients with bipolar disorder are 10 times more likely to develop the illness.
- Concordance rates for monozygotic twins are 40–70%, and rates for dizygotic twins range from 5 to 25%.
- Bipolar I has the highest genetic link of all major psychiatric disorders.

Course and Prognosis

- Untreated manic episodes generally last several months.
- The course is usually chronic with relapses; as the disease progresses, episodes may occur more frequently.
- Ninety percent of individuals after one manic episode will have a repeat mood episode within 5 years.

- Bipolar disorder has a poorer prognosis than MDD.
- Maintenance treatment with mood stabilizing medications between episodes helps to ↓ the risk of relapse.
- Twenty-five to 50% of people with bipolar disorder attempt suicide, and 10–15% die by suicide.

Treatment

- **Pharmacotherapy:**
  - Lithium is a mood stabilizer; 50–70% treated with lithium show partial reduction of mania. Long-term use **reduces suicide risk**. Acute overdose can be fatal due to its low therapeutic index.
  - The anticonvulsants carbamazepine and valproic acid are also mood stabilizers. They are particularly useful for rapid cycling bipolar disorder and those with mixed features.
  - Atypical antipsychotics (risperidone, olanzapine, quetiapine, ziprasidone) are effective as both monotherapy and adjunct therapy for acute mania. In fact, many patients (especially with severe mania and/or with psychotic features) are treated with a combination of a mood stabilizer and antipsychotic; studies have shown a greater and faster response with combination therapy.
  - Antidepressants are discouraged as monotherapy due to concerns of activating mania or hypomania. They are occasionally used to treat depressive episodes when patients concurrently take mood stabilizers.
- **Psychotherapy:** Supportive psychotherapy, family therapy, group therapy (may prolong remission once the acute manic episode has been controlled).
- **ECT:**
  - Works well in treatment of manic episodes.
  - Some patients require more treatments (up to 20) than for depression.
  - Especially effective for refractory or life-threatening acute mania or depression.

BIPOLAR II DISORDER

Alternatively called **recurrent major depressive episodes with hypomania.**

Diagnosis and DSM-5 Criteria

History of one or more major depressive episodes and at least one **hypomanic** episode. *Remember:* If there has been a full manic episode, *even in the past*, then the diagnosis is bipolar I, *not* bipolar II disorder.

Epidemiology

- Prevalence is unclear, with some studies > and others < than bipolar I.
- May be slightly more common in women.
- Onset usually before age 30.
- No ethnic differences seen.
- Frequently misdiagnosed as unipolar depression and thereby inappropriately treated.

Etiology

Same as bipolar I disorder (see above).

WARDS TIP

Side effects of lithium include:
- Weight gain
- Tremor
- Gastrointestinal disturbances
- Fatigue
- Cardiac arrhythmias
- Seizures
- Goiter/hypothyroidism
- Leukocytosis (benign)
- Coma (in toxic doses)
- Polyuria (nephrogenic diabetes insipidus)
- Polydipsia
- Alopecia
- Metallic taste

KEY FACT

ECT is the best treatment for a pregnant woman who is having a manic episode. It provides a good alternative to antipsychotics and can be used with relative safety in all trimesters.

KEY FACT

Treatment for bipolar disorder includes lithium, valproic acid, and carbamazepine (for rapid cyclers), or second-generation antipsychotics. Lithium remains the gold standard, particularly due to demonstrated reduction in suicide risk.

KEY FACT

A patient with a history of postpartum mania has a high risk of relapse with future deliveries and should be treated with mood stabilizing agents as prophylaxis. However, some of these medications may be contraindicated in breast-feeding.

Course and Prognosis

Tends to be chronic, requiring long-term treatment. Likely better prognosis than bipolar I.

Treatment

Fewer studies focus on the treatment for bipolar II. Currently, treatment is the same as bipolar I disorder (see above).

SPECIFIERS FOR BIPOLAR DISORDERS

- **Anxious distress:** Defined by feeling keyed up/tense, restless, difficulty concentrating, fears of something bad happening, and feelings of loss of control.
- **Mixed features:** Depressive symptoms present during the majority of days during mania/hypomania: dysphoria/depressed mood, anhedonia, psychomotor retardation, fatigue/loss of energy, feelings of worthlessness or inappropriate guilt, thoughts of death or suicidal ideation.
- **Rapid cycling:** At least four mood episodes (manic, hypomanic, depressed) within 12 months.
- **Melancholic features** (*during depressed episode*): Characterized by *anhedonia*, early morning awakenings, depression worse in the morning, psychomotor disturbance, excessive guilt, and anorexia.
- **Atypical features** (*during depressed episode*): Characterized by hypersomnia, hyperphagia, reactive mood, leaden paralysis, and hypersensitivity to interpersonal rejection.
- **Psychotic features:** Characterized by the presence of delusions and/or hallucinations.
- **Catatonia:** Catalepsy, purposeless motor activity, extreme negativism or mutism, bizarre postures, and echolalia. Especially responsive to ECT.
- **Peripartum onset:** Onset of manic or hypomanic symptoms occurs during pregnancy or 4 weeks following delivery.
- **Seasonal pattern:** Temporal relationship between onset of mania/hypomania and particular time of the year.

PERSISTENT DEPRESSIVE DISORDER (DYSTHYMIA)

Patients with persistent depressive disorder (dysthymia) have chronic depression most of the time, and they may have discrete major depressive episodes.

Diagnosis and DSM-5 Criteria

1. Depressed mood for the majority of time most days for at least 2 years (in children or adolescents for at least 1 year)
2. At least two of the following:
   - Poor concentration or difficulty making decisions
   - Feelings of hopelessness
   - Poor appetite or overeating
   - Insomnia or hypersomnia
   - Low energy or fatigue
   - Low self-esteem
3. During the 2-year period:
   - The person has not been without the above symptoms for >2 months at a time.

- May have major depressive episode(s) or meet criteria for major depression continuously.
- The patient must never have had a manic or hypomanic episode (this would make the diagnosis bipolar disorder or cyclothymic disorder, respectively).

Epidemiology

- 12-month prevalence: 2%.
- More common in women.
- Onset often in childhood, adolescence, and early adulthood.

Course and Prognosis

Early and insidious onset, with a chronic course. Depressive symptoms much less likely to resolve than in MDD.

Treatment

- Combination treatment with psychotherapy and pharmacotherapy is more efficacious than either alone.
- Cognitive therapy, interpersonal therapy, and insight-oriented psychotherapy are the most effective.
- Antidepressants found to be beneficial include SSRIs, TCAs, and MAOIs.

CYCLOTHYMIC DISORDER

Alternating periods of hypomania and periods with mild-to-moderate depressive symptoms.

Diagnosis and DSM-5 Criteria

- Numerous periods with hypomanic symptoms (but not a full hypomanic episode) and periods with depressive symptoms (but not full MDE) for at least 2 years.
- The person must never have been symptom free for >2 months during those 2 years.
- No history of major depressive episode, hypomania, or manic episode.

Epidemiology

- Lifetime prevalence: <1%.
- May coexist with borderline personality disorder.
- Onset usually age 15–25.
- Occurs equally in males and females.

Course and Prognosis

Chronic course; approximately one-third of patients eventually develop bipolar I/II disorder.

Treatment

Antimanic agents (mood stabilizers or second-generation antipsychotics) as used to treat bipolar disorder (see above).

PREMENSTRUAL DYSPHORIC DISORDER

Mood lability, irritability, dysphoria, and anxiety that occur repeatedly during the premenstrual phase of the cycle.

Diagnosis and DSM-5 Criteria

- In most menstrual cycles, at least five symptoms are present: in the final week before menses, improve within a few days after menses, and are minimal/absent in the week postmenses (should be confirmed by daily ratings for at least 2 menstrual cycles).
- At least one of the following symptoms is present: affective lability, irritability/anger, depressed mood, anxiety/tension.
- At least one of the following symptoms is present (for total of at least five symptoms when combined with above): anhedonia, problems concentrating, anergia, appetite changes/food cravings, hypersomnia/insomnia, feeling overwhelmed/out of control, physical symptoms (e.g., breast tenderness/swelling, joint/muscle pain, bloating, weight gain).
- Symptoms cause clinically significant distress or impairment in functioning.
- Symptoms are not only exacerbation of another disorder (e.g., MDD, panic disorder, persistent depressive disorder).
- Symptoms are not due to a substance (medication or drug) or another medical condition.

Epidemiology/Etiology

- Prevalence: 1.8%.
- Onset can occur at any time after menarche.
- Has been observed worldwide.
- Environmental and genetic factors contribute.

Course and Prognosis

Symptoms may worsen prior to menopause but cease after menopause.

Treatment

SSRIs are first-line treatment, either as daily therapy or luteal phase-only treatment (starting on cycle day 14 and stopping upon menses or shortly thereafter). Oral contraceptives may reduce symptoms. Gonadotropin-releasing hormone (GnRH) agonists have also been used, and, in rare cases, bilateral oophorectomy with hysterectomy will resolve symptoms.

DISRUPTIVE MOOD DYSREGULATION DISORDER (DMDD)

Chronic, severe, persistent irritability occurring in childhood and adolescence.

Diagnosis and DSM-5 Criteria

- Severe recurrent verbal and/or physical outbursts out of proportion to situation.
- Outbursts ≥3 per week and inconsistent with developmental level.
- Mood between outbursts is persistently angry/irritable most of the day nearly every day, and is observed by others.
- Symptoms for at least 1 year, and no more than 3 months without symptoms.
- Symptoms in at least 2 settings (e.g., home, school, peers).
- Symptoms must have started before age 10, but diagnosis can be made from ages 6 to 18.
- No episodes meeting full criteria for manic/hypomanic episode lasting longer than 1 day.

- Behaviors do not occur during MDD and not better explained by another mental disorder (this disorder cannot coexist with oppositional defiant disorder, intermittent explosive disorder, or bipolar disorder).
- Symptoms not due to a substance (medication or drug) or another medical condition.

Epidemiology/Etiology

- Prevalence is unclear as this is a new diagnosis.
- 6–12-month prevalence rates of chronic/severe persistent irritability in children: 2–5%.
- Rates likely greater in males than females.

Course and Prognosis

- By definition DMDD must occur prior to 10 years.
- Approximately 50% of those with DMDD continue to meet criteria after 1 year.
- Rates of conversion to bipolar disorder are very low.
- Very high rates of comorbidity, especially with ODD, ADHD, mood disorders, and anxiety disorders.

Treatment

- Given the new nature of this disorder, there are no consensus evidenced-based treatments. Psychotherapy, such as parent management training, for the patient and family is generally first line.
- Medications should be used to treat comorbid disorders.
- Stimulants, SSRIs, mood stabilizers, and second-generation antipsychotics have all been used to treat the primary symptoms of DMDD.

OTHER DISORDERS OF MOOD IN DSM-5

- Mood disorder due to another medical condition.
- Substance/Medication-induced mood disorder.
- Specified depressive/bipolar disorder (meets criteria for MDE or bipolar except shorter duration or too few symptoms)
- Unspecified depressive/bipolar disorder

CHAPTER 5

ANXIETY, OBSESSIVE-COMPULSIVE, TRAUMA, AND STRESSOR-RELATED DISORDERS

Pharmacotherapy   49

Psychotherapy   49
    PANIC ATTACKS   49

Anxiety Disorders   50
    PANIC DISORDER   50
    AGORAPHOBIA   51
    SPECIFIC PHOBIAS/SOCIAL ANXIETY DISORDER (SOCIAL PHOBIA)   51
    SELECTIVE MUTISM   52
    SEPARATION ANXIETY DISORDER   53
    GENERALIZED ANXIETY DISORDER (GAD)   54

Obsessive-Compulsive and Related Disorders   55
    OBSESSIVE-COMPULSIVE DISORDER (OCD)   55
    BODY DYSMORPHIC DISORDER   56
    HOARDING DISORDER   57
    TRICHOTILLOMANIA (HAIR-PULLING DISORDER)   57
    EXCORIATION (SKIN-PICKING) DISORDER   58

Trauma and Stressor-Related Disorders   58
    POSTTRAUMATIC STRESS DISORDER (PTSD) AND
    ACUTE STRESS DISORDER   59
    ADJUSTMENT DISORDERS   60

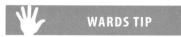

WARDS TIP

Assess for psychopathology based on if the patient's symptoms are causing **S**ocial and/or **O**ccupational **D**ysfunction **(SOD).**

WARDS TIP

Late-onset anxiety symptoms without prior or family psychiatric history should increase suspicion of anxiety caused by another medical condition or substance.

Anxiety is defined as an individual's emotional and physical fear response to a perceived threat. Pathologic anxiety occurs when the symptoms are **excessive, irrational, out of proportion to the trigger** or are **without an identifiable trigger**. Maladaptive anxiety **persists longer** and feels more intense than transient, situational anxiety (Table 5-1). The **criteria for most anxiety disorders involve symptoms that cause clinically significant distress or impairment in social and/or occupational functioning.**

- Anxiety disorders are caused by a combination of genetic, biological, environmental, and psychosocial factors.
- Primary anxiety disorders can only be diagnosed after determining that the signs and symptoms are **NOT due to the physiological effects of a substance, medication** (see Table 5-2), **or medical condition** (see Table 5-3).
- Major neurotransmitter systems implicated: norepinephrine (NE), serotonin (5-HT), and gamma-aminobutyric acid (GABA)
- **Most common form of psychopathology**
- **Lifetime prevalence: women 30%, men 19%**
- **More frequently seen in women** compared to men, about 2:1 ratio

Treatment guidelines
- Based on the level of symptom impairment, consider **psychotherapy for milder** presentations while initiating **combination treatment** with **pharmacotherapy for moderate to severe** anxiety.

TABLE 5-1.   Signs and Symptoms of Anxiety

Constitutional	Fatigue, diaphoresis, shivering
Cardiac	Chest pain, palpitations, tachycardia, hypertension
Pulmonary	Shortness of breath, hyperventilation
Neurologic/ Musculoskeletal	Vertigo, lightheadedness, paresthesias, tremors, insomnia, muscle tension
Gastrointestinal	Abdominal discomfort, anorexia, nausea, emesis, diarrhea, constipation

TABLE 5-2.   Medications and Substances That Cause Anxiety

Alcohol	Intoxication/withdrawal
Sedatives, hypnotics or anxiolytics	Withdrawal
Cannabis	Intoxication
Hallucinogens (PCP, LSD, MDMA)	Intoxication
Stimulants (amphetamines, cocaine)	Intoxication/withdrawal
Caffeine	Intoxication
Tobacco	Intoxication/withdrawal
Opioids	Withdrawal

Note: PCP, phencyclidine; LSD, lysergic acid diethylamide; MDMA, 3,4-methylenedioxy methamphetamine.

TABLE 5-3.   Medical Conditions That Cause Anxiety

Neurologic	Epilepsy, migraines, brain tumors, multiple sclerosis, Huntington's disease
Endocrine	Hyperthyroidism, thyrotoxicosis, hypoglycemia, pheochromocytoma, carcinoid syndrome
Metabolic	Vitamin B_{12} deficiency, electrolyte abnormalities, porphyria
Respiratory	Asthma, chronic obstructive pulmonary disease (COPD), hypoxia, pulmonary embolism (PE), pneumonia, pneumothorax
Cardiovascular	Congestive heart failure (CHF), angina, arrhythmia, myocardial infarction (MI)

Pharmacotherapy

- **First-line:** Selective serotonin reuptake inhibitors (**SSRIs**) (e.g., sertraline) and serotonin-norepinephrine reuptake inhibitors (SNRIs) (e.g., venlafaxine)
  - **Benzodiazepines** (enhance activity of GABA at GABA-A receptor) work quickly and effectively, but they all can be addictive. Minimize the use, duration, and dose. Benzodiazepines should be avoided in patients with a history of substance use disorders, particularly alcohol.
  - Consider nonaddicting anxiolytic alternatives for PRN use, such as diphenhydramine or hydroxyzine.
  - **Buspirone**, a 5-HT$_{1A}$ partial agonist, is a non-benzodiazepine anxiolytic; however, it is not commonly used due to minimal efficacy and often only prescribed as augmentation.
  - **Beta-blockers (e.g., propranolol)** may be used to help control autonomic symptoms (e.g., palpitations, tachycardia, sweating) with **panic attacks** or **performance anxiety**.
  - **Tricyclic antidepressants** (TCAs) and **monoamine oxidase inhibitors** (MAOIs) may be considered if first-line agents are not effective. Their side-effect profile makes them less tolerable.

Psychotherapy

- Many modalities of psychotherapy are helpful for patients suffering from anxiety disorders.
  - **Cognitive behavioral therapy (CBT)** has been proven effective for anxiety disorders. CBT examines the relationship between anxiety-driven cognitions (thoughts), emotions, and behavior.
  - **Psychodynamic psychotherapy** facilitates understanding and insight into the development of anxiety and ultimately increases anxiety tolerance.

PANIC ATTACKS

Panic attacks are a type of fear response involving an abrupt surge of intense anxiety which may be triggered or occur spontaneously. Panic attacks peak

---

WARDS TIP

SSRIs typically take about 4–6 weeks to become fully effective, and higher doses (than used in treating depression) are generally required.

KEY FACT

If a patient has a comorbid depressive disorder, consider alternatives to benzodiazepines as they may worsen depression.

WARDS TIP

Use *benzodiazepines* to temporarily *bridge* patients until long-term medication becomes effective.

WARDS TIP

Use the *Bs* to *Block* the *Ps*: *Beta-Blockers* for *Panic* attacks and *Performance* anxiety.

WARDS TIP

Pharmacologic goal: achieve symptomatic relief and continue treatment for at least 6 months before attempting to titrate off medications.

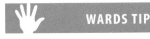

WARDS TIP

Medications can reduce symptoms enough so that a patient can participate in therapy. Therapy can help prevent relapse if medications are no longer prescribed.

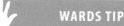

KEY FACT

Symptoms of panic attacks
Da PANICS

Dizziness, **d**isconnectedness, **d**erealization (unreality), **d**epersonalization (detached from self)

Palpitations, **p**aresthesias

Abdominal distress

Numbness, **n**ausea

Intense fear of dying, losing control or "going crazy"

Chills, **c**hest pain

Sweating, **s**haking, **s**hortness of breath

WARDS TIP

Smoking is a risk factor for panic attacks.

KEY FACT

When a patient presents with a panic attack, rule out potentially life-threatening medical conditions such as a heart attack, thyrotoxicosis, and thromboembolism.

WARDS TIP

A classic example of a panic disorder case: a woman with no medical history who repeatedly visits the ER with episodes of palpitations, diaphoresis, and shortness of breath. Because of these cardiopulmonary symptoms, she fears that she is dying. Her medical workup is negative.

WARDS TIP

Carefully screen patients with panic attacks for suicidality—they are at an increased risk for suicide attempts.

within minutes and usually resolve within half an hour. Patients may continue to feel anxious for hours afterwards and confuse this for a prolonged panic attack. Although classically associated with panic disorder, panic attacks can also be experienced with other anxiety disorders, psychiatric disorders, and other medical conditions.

Anxiety Disorders

PANIC DISORDER

Panic disorder is characterized by *spontaneous*, recurrent panic attacks. These attacks occur suddenly, *"out of the blue."* Patients may also experience panic attacks with a clear trigger. The frequency of attacks ranges from multiple times per day to a few monthly. Patients develop debilitating anticipatory anxiety about having future attacks—"fear of the fear." This can lead to avoidance behaviors and become so severe as to leave patients homebound (i.e., *agoraphobia*).

Diagnosis and DSM-5 Criteria

- **Recurrent, *unexpected* panic attacks** without an identifiable trigger
- One or more of panic attacks followed by ≥1 month of continuous worry about experiencing subsequent attacks or their consequences, and/or a maladaptive change in behaviors (e.g., avoidance of possible triggers)
- Not caused by the direct effects of a substance, another mental disorder, or another medical condition

Etiology

- Genetic factors: Greater risk of panic disorder if first-degree relative affected
- Psychosocial factors: ↑ incidence of stressors (especially loss) prior to onset of disorder; history of childhood physical or sexual abuse

Epidemiology

- Lifetime prevalence: 4%
- Higher rates in woman compared to men about 2:1
- Median age of onset: 20–24 years old

Course and Prognosis

- Panic disorder has a chronic course with waxing and waning symptoms. Relapses are common with discontinuation of medical therapy.
- Only a minority of patients has full remission of symptoms.
- Up to 65% of patients with panic disorder have major depression.
- Other comorbid syndromes include other anxiety disorders (especially agoraphobia), bipolar disorder, and alcohol use disorder.

Treatment

Pharmacotherapy and CBT—most effective
- First-line: **SSRIs** (e.g., sertraline, citalopram, escitalopram)
- Can switch to TCAs (clomipramine, imipramine) if SSRIs not effective
- Can use benzodiazepines (clonazepam, lorazepam) as scheduled or PRN (as needed), especially until the other medications reach full efficacy.

AGORAPHOBIA

Agoraphobia is intense fear of being in public places where escape or obtaining help may be difficult. It often develops with panic disorder. The course of the disorder is usually chronic. Avoidance behaviors may become as extreme as complete confinement to the home.

Diagnosis and DSM-5 Criteria

- Intense fear/anxiety about >2 situations due to concern of difficulty escaping or obtaining help in case of panic or other humiliating symptoms:
    - outside of the home alone
    - open spaces (e.g., bridges)
    - enclosed places (e.g., stores)
    - public transportation (e.g., trains)
    - crowds/lines
- The triggering situations cause fear/anxiety out of proportion to the potential danger posed, leading to endurance of intense anxiety, avoidance, or requiring a companion. This holds true even if the patient suffers from a medical condition such as inflammatory bowel disease (IBS) which may lead to embarrassing public scenarios.
- Symptoms cause significant social or occupational dysfunction
- Symptoms last ≥ 6 months
- Symptoms not better explained by another mental disorder

Etiology

- Strong genetic factor: Heritability about 60%
- Psychosocial factor: Onset frequently follows a traumatic event

Course/Prognosis

- >50% of patients experience a panic attack prior to developing agoraphobia
- Onset is usually before age 35
- Course is persistent and chronic, with rare full remission
- Comorbid diagnoses include other anxiety disorders, depressive disorders, and substance use disorders

Treatment

- Similar approach as panic disorder: CBT and SSRIs (for panic symptoms)

SPECIFIC PHOBIAS/SOCIAL ANXIETY DISORDER (SOCIAL PHOBIA)

A phobia is defined as an **irrational fear that leads to endurance of the anxiety and/or avoidance** of the feared object or situation. A *specific phobia* is **an intense fear of a specific object or situation** (i.e., the phobic stimulus). *Social anxiety disorder (social phobia)* is the **fear of scrutiny by others or fear of acting in a humiliating or embarrassing way**. The phobia may develop in the wake of negative or traumatic encounters with the stimulus. Social situations causing significant anxiety may be avoided altogether, resulting in social and academic/occupational impairment.

Diagnosis and DSM-5 Criteria

- Persistent, excessive fear elicited by a specific situation or object which is out of proportion to any actual danger/threat
- Exposure to the situation triggers an immediate fear response

- Situation or object is avoided when possible or tolerated with intense anxiety
- Symptoms cause significant social or occupational dysfunction
- Duration ≥6 months
- Symptoms not solely due to another mental disorder, substance (medication or drug), or another medical condition

The diagnostic criteria for **social anxiety disorder (social phobia)** are similar to the above except the phobic stimulus is related to social scrutiny and negative evaluation. The patients fear embarrassment, humiliation, and rejection. This fear may be limited to performance or public speaking, which may be routinely encountered in the patient's occupation or academic pursuit.

Epidemiology

- Phobias are the **most common psychiatric disorder** in women and **second most common in men** (substance-related is first)
- Lifetime prevalence of specific phobia: >10%
- Mean age of onset for specific phobia is 10 years old; median age of onset for social anxiety disorder is 13 years old
- Specific phobia rates are higher in women compared to men (2:1) but vary depending on the type of stimulus
- Social anxiety disorder occurs equally in men and women

Treatment

Specific phobia:
- Treatment of choice: CBT

Social anxiety disorder (social phobia):
- Treatment of choice: CBT
- First-line medication, if needed: SSRIs (e.g., sertraline, fluoxetine) or SNRI (e.g., venlafaxine) for debilitating symptoms
- Benzodiazepines (e.g., clonazepam, lorazepam) can be used as scheduled or PRN
- **Beta-blockers** (e.g., atenolol, **propranolol**) for performance anxiety/public speaking

SELECTIVE MUTISM

Selective mutism is a rare condition characterized by a failure to speak in specific situations for at least 1 month, despite the intact ability to comprehend and use language. Symptom onset typically starts during childhood. The majority of these patients suffer from anxiety, particularly social anxiety as the mutism manifests in social settings. The patients may remain completely silent or whisper. They may use nonverbal means of communication, such as writing or gesturing. While communication delays or disorders may co-occur, they would not account for the selective mutism.

Diagnosis and DSM-5 Criteria

- Consistent failure to speak in select social situations (e.g., school) despite speech ability in other scenarios
- Mutism is not due to a language difficulty or a communication disorder
- Symptoms cause significant impairment in academic, occupational, or social functioning
- Symptoms last >1 month (extending beyond 1st month of school)

Treatment

- Psychotherapy: CBT, family therapy
- Medications: SSRIs for anxiety (especially with comorbid social anxiety disorder)

SEPARATION ANXIETY DISORDER

As part of normal human development, infants become distressed when they are separated from their primary caregiver. *Stranger anxiety* begins around 6 months and peaks around 9 months, while *separation anxiety* typically emerges by 1 year old and peaks by 18 months. When the anxiety due to separation becomes extreme or developmentally inappropriate, it is considered pathologic. Separation anxiety disorder may be preceded by a stressful life event.

Diagnosis and DSM-5 Criteria

- **Excessive and developmentally inappropriate fear/anxiety** regarding **separation from attachment figures**, with at least three of the following:
- Separation from attachment figures leads to extreme distress.
- Excessive worry about loss of or harm to attachment figures.
- Excessive worry about experiencing an event that leads to separation from attachment figures.
- Reluctance to leave home, or attend school or work.
- Reluctance to be alone.
- Reluctance to sleep alone or away from home.
- Complaints of physical symptoms when separated from major attachment figures.
- Nightmares of separation and refusal to sleep without proximity to attachment figure.
- Lasts for ≥4 weeks in children/adolescents and ≥6 months in adults.
- Symptoms cause significant social, academic, or occupational dysfunction.
- Symptoms not due to another mental disorder.

Treatment

- Psychotherapy: CBT, family therapy
- Medications: SSRIs can be effective as an adjunct to therapy

> **WARDS TIP**
>
> Separation anxiety may lead to complaints of somatic symptoms to avoid school/work.

Ms. Johnson is a 24-year-old law student who presents to an outpatient psychiatry clinic accompanied by her husband. She feels "worried about everything!" She is "stressed out" about her academic workload and upcoming exams. She feels fatigued and has difficulty concentrating on her assignments. She also complains of frequent headaches and associated neck muscle spasms, as well as difficulty falling asleep.

The patient's husband describes her as "a worrier. She'll worry about me getting into an accident, losing my job, not making enough money—the list goes on and on."

Ms. Johnson reports that she has always had some degree of anxiety, but previously found that it motivated her. Over the last year, her symptoms have become debilitating and beyond her control.

What is Ms. Johnson's most likely diagnosis?

Her most likely diagnosis is generalized anxiety disorder (GAD). The key point in identifying her diagnosis is her history of *excessive worrying* about *everything*. Like many patients with GAD, she is described as a "*worrier*." She reports typical associated symptoms: insomnia, fatigue, muscle tension, and impaired concentration. Her symptoms have been present for over *6 months*.

What is the next step?

A complete physical exam and medical workup should be performed in order to rule out other medical conditions or substance use contributing to or causing her anxiety symptoms.

What are Ms. Johnson's treatment options?

Treatment options for GAD include psychotherapy (usually CBT) and pharmacotherapy (typically SSRIs). A combination of both modalities may achieve better remission rates than either treatment alone.

WARDS TIP

GAD Mnemonic
Worry WARTS
Worried
Wound up, **w**orn-out
Absent-minded
Restless
Tense
Sleepless

WARDS TIP

For patients with anxiety, evaluate for caffeine use and recommend significant reduction or elimination.

WARDS TIP

Exercise can significantly reduce anxiety.

GENERALIZED ANXIETY DISORDER (GAD)

Patients with GAD have persistent, excessive anxiety about many aspects of their daily lives. Often, they experience somatic symptoms including fatigue and muscle tension. Not uncommonly, these physical complaints lead patients to initially present to a primary care physician. GAD is highly comorbid with other anxiety and depressive disorders.

Diagnosis and DSM-5 Criteria

- Excessive, anxiety/worry about various daily events/activities ≥6 months
- Difficulty controlling the worry
- Associated ≥3 symptoms: restlessness, fatigue, impaired concentration, irritability, muscle tension, insomnia
- Symptoms are not caused by the direct effects of a substance, or another mental disorder or medical condition
- Symptoms cause significant social or occupational dysfunction

Epidemiology/Etiology

- Lifetime prevalence: 5–9%
- GAD rates higher in women compared to men (2:1)
- 1/3 of risk for developing GAD is genetic

Course/Prognosis

- Symptoms of worry begin in childhood
- Median age of onset of GAD: 30 years old
- Course is chronic, with waxing and waning symptoms
- Rates of full remission are low
- Comorbid diagnoses include other anxiety disorders and depressive disorders

Treatment

The most effective treatment approach combines psychotherapy and pharmacotherapy:

- CBT
- SSRI (e.g., sertraline, citalopram) or SNRI (e.g., venlafaxine)
- Can also consider a short-term course of benzodiazepines or augmentation with buspirone
- Much less commonly used medications are TCAs and MAOIs

Obsessive-Compulsive and Related Disorders

OBSESSIVE-COMPULSIVE DISORDER (OCD)

OCD is characterized by obsessions and/or compulsions that are time-consuming, distressing, and impairing. **Obsessions** are recurrent, intrusive, undesired thoughts that ↑ anxiety. Patients may attempt to relieve this anxiety by performing **compulsions**, which are repetitive behaviors or mental rituals. Anxiety may increase when a patient resists acting out a compulsion.

Patients with OCD have varying degrees of insight.

Diagnosis and DSM-5 Criteria

- Experiencing obsessions and/or compulsions that are time-consuming (e.g., >1 hour/daily) or cause significant distress or dysfunction
  - **Obsessions:** Recurrent, intrusive, anxiety-provoking thoughts, images, or urges that the patient attempts to suppress, ignore, or neutralize by some other thought or action (i.e., by performing a compulsion)
  - **Compulsions:** Repetitive behaviors or mental acts the patient feels driven to perform in response to an obsession or a rule aimed at stress reduction or disaster prevention. The behaviors are not realistically linked with what they are to prevent or are excessive.
- Not caused by the direct effects of a substance, another mental illness, or another medical condition

Epidemiology

- Lifetime prevalence: 2–3%
- Mean age of onset: 20 years old
- No gender difference in prevalence overall

Etiology

- Significant genetic component: Higher rates of OCD in first-degree relatives and monozygotic twins than in the general population. Higher rate of OCD in first-degree relatives with Tourette's disorder.

Course/Prognosis

- Chronic, with waxing and waning symptoms
- <20% remission rate without treatment
- Suicidal ideation in 50%, attempts in 25% of patients with OCD
- High comorbidity with other anxiety disorders (>75%), depressive or bipolar disorder (>60%), obsessive-compulsive personality disorder (up to 32%), and tic disorder (up to 30%)

WARDS TIP

As the name suggests, the worries associated with *generalized* anxiety disorder are free-floating across various areas, as opposed to being fixed on a specific trigger.

KEY FACT

Compulsions can often take the form of repeated checking or counting.

KEY FACT

Patients with OCD often initially seek help from primary care and other nonpsychiatric providers for help with the consequences of compulsions (e.g., excessive washing).

KEY FACT

The triad of "uncontrollable urges"— OCD, ADHD, and tic disorder—are usually first seen in children or adolescents.

KEY FACT

Common Patterns of Obsessions and Compulsions

Obsessions	Compulsions
Contamination	Cleaning or avoidance of contaminant
Doubt or harm (e.g., oven on)	Checking multiple times to avoid potential danger
Symmetry	Ordering or counting
Intrusive, taboo thoughts (e.g., sexual, violent)	With or without related compulsion

Treatment

Utilize a combination of psychopharmacology and CBT

CBT focuses on *exposure and response prevention*: prolonged, graded exposure to ritual-eliciting stimulus and prevention of the relieving compulsion

- First-line medication: SSRIs (e.g., sertraline, fluoxetine), typically at higher doses
- Can also use the most serotonin selective **TCA, Clomipramine**
- Can augment with atypical antipsychotics
- **Last resort:** In treatment-resistant, severely debilitating cases, can use psychosurgery (cingulotomy) or electroconvulsive therapy (ECT) (especially if comorbid depression is present).

BODY DYSMORPHIC DISORDER

- Patients with body dysmorphic disorder are preoccupied with body parts that they perceive as flawed or defective, having strong beliefs that they are unattractive or repulsive.
- Though their physical imperfections are either minimal or not observable, patients view them as severe and grotesque.
- They spend significant time trying to correct perceived flaws with makeup, dermatological procedures, or plastic surgery.

Diagnosis and DSM-5 Criteria

- Preoccupation with one or more perceived defects or flaws in physical appearance that are not observable by or appear slight to others
- Repetitive behaviors (e.g., skin picking, excessive grooming) or mental acts (e.g., comparing appearance to others) are performed in response to the appearance concerns
- Preoccupation causes significant distress or impairment in functioning
- Appearance preoccupation is not better accounted for by concerns with body fat/weight in an eating disorder

Epidemiology

- May be slightly more common in women than men
- Prevalence elevated in those with high rates of childhood abuse and neglect, as well as in first-degree relatives of patients with OCD
- Higher prevalence in dermatologic and cosmetic surgery patients
- Mean age of onset: 15 years old

Course/Prognosis

- The onset is usually gradual, beginning in early adolescence. Symptoms tend to be chronic.
- Surgical or dermatological procedures are routinely unsuccessful in satisfying the patient.
- High rate of suicidal ideation and attempts
- Comorbidity with major depression, social anxiety disorder (social phobia), and OCD

Treatment

- SSRIs and/or CBT may reduce the obsessive and compulsive symptoms in many patients.

KEY FACT

Although similar sounding with superficial resemblance, OCD and obsessive-compulsive personality disorder (OCPD) have distinct presentations. Individuals with OCPD are obsessed with details, control, and perfectionism; they are not intruded upon by unwanted preoccupations nor compelled to carry out compulsions. OCD patients are *dis*tressed by their symptoms (ego-*dys*tonic); OCPD patients do not perceive them as an *issue* (ego-*syn*tonic).

HOARDING DISORDER

Diagnosis and DSM-5 Criteria

- Persistent difficulty discarding possessions, regardless of value.
- Difficulty is due to need to save the items and distress associated with discarding them.
- Results in accumulation of possessions that congest/clutter living areas and compromise use.
- Hoarding causes clinically significant distress or impairment in social, occupational, or other areas of functioning.
- Hoarding is not attributable to another medical condition or another mental disorder.

Epidemiology/Etiology

- Unclear lifetime prevalence but point prevalence of significant hoarding is 2–6%.
- Unclear gender preference.
- Hoarding 3× more prevalent in older population.
- Individuals with hoarding often report stressful and traumatic events preceding the onset of hoarding.
- Large genetic component, with 50% of individuals with hoarding having a relative who also hoards.

Course/Prognosis

- Hoarding behavior begins in early teens.
- Hoarding tends to worsen.
- Usually chronic course.
- 75% of individuals have comorbid mood (MDD) or anxiety disorder (social anxiety disorder).
- 20% of individuals have comorbid OCD.

Treatment

- Very difficult to treat.
- Specialized CBT for hoarding.
- SSRIs can be used, but not as beneficial unless OCD symptoms are present.

TRICHOTILLOMANIA (HAIR-PULLING DISORDER)

Diagnosis and DSM-5 Criteria

- Recurrent pulling out of one's hair, resulting in hair loss.
- Repeated attempts to decrease or stop hair pulling.
- Causes significant distress or impairment in daily functioning.
- Hair pulling or hair loss is not due to another medical condition or psychiatric disorder.
- Usually involves the scalp, eyebrows, or eyelashes, but may include facial, axillary, and pubic hair.

Epidemiology/Etiology

- Lifetime prevalence: 1–2% of the adult population.
- More common in women than in men (10:1 ratio).

- Onset usually at the time of puberty and frequently associated with a stressful event.
- Site of hair pulling may vary, and specific hair textures may be preferred.
- Etiology may involve biological, genetic, and environmental factors.
- ↑ incidence of comorbid OCD, major depressive disorder, and excoriation (skin-picking) disorder.
- Course may be chronic with waxing and waning periods; adult onset is generally more difficult to treat.

Treatment

- Treatment includes medications such as SSRIs, second-generation antipsychotics, N-acetylcysteine, or lithium.
- Forms of cognitive-behavior therapy (e.g., habit reversal training) are the best-evidenced psychotherapy.

EXCORIATION (SKIN-PICKING) DISORDER

Diagnosis and DSM-5 Criteria

- Recurrent skin picking resulting in lesions.
- Repeated attempts to decrease or stop skin picking.
- Causes significant distress or impairment in daily functioning.
- Skin picking is not due to a substance, another medical condition, or another psychiatric disorder.

Epidemiology/Etiology

- Lifetime prevalence: 1.4% of the adult population.
- >75% of cases are women.
- More common in individuals with OCD and first-degree family members.

Course/Prognosis

- Skin picking begins in adolescence.
- Course is chronic, with waxing and waning periods if untreated.
- Comorbidity with OCD, trichotillomania, and MDD.

Treatment

- Treatment is similar to that for trichotillomania.
- Specialized types of cognitive-behavior therapy (e.g., habit reversal training).
- SSRIs have also shown some benefit.

Trauma and Stressor-Related Disorders

A 19-year-old freshman is brought to the ER by her college dorm mate. The dorm mate reports that the patient has been isolating herself, crying in their room, and screaming in her sleep. The dorm mate states, "this isn't like her at all" and discloses concern that something happened at a recent party they attended 5 weeks ago. "She hasn't been the same since." The patient is reluctant to talk at first but eventually admits that at that party she was forced to have sex with one of the fraternity brothers. She hazily recalls the details and the aftermath. Ever since then, she has felt "horrible." She describes intrusive thoughts and nightmares. The patient feels constantly on edge and is afraid she will be victimized again. She has avoided most places where she might encounter the rapist and felt safest not leaving the dorm room. Her sense of shame and embarrassment have kept her emotionally isolated, and her symptoms have resulted in her grades dropping.

What is the most likely diagnosis?

After being a victim of sexual violence, the patient has been suffering from symptoms consistent with PTSD for the last 5 weeks: reliving the trauma via intrusive thoughts and nightmares, avoidance of the attacker, hypervigilance, and negative mood.

POSTTRAUMATIC STRESS DISORDER (PTSD) AND ACUTE STRESS DISORDER

PTSD is characterized by the development of multiple symptoms after exposure to one or more traumatic events: intrusive symptoms (e.g., nightmares, flashbacks), avoidance, negative alterations in thoughts and mood, and increased arousal. The symptoms last for at least a month and may occur immediately after the trauma or with delayed expression.

Acute Stress Disorder is diagnosed in patients who experience a major traumatic event and suffer from similar symptoms as PTSD (see Table 5-4) but for a shorter duration. The onset of symptoms occurs within 1 month of the trauma and symptoms last for less than 1 month.

Diagnosis and DSM-5 Criteria

- Exposure to actual or threatened death, serious injury, or sexual violence by directly experiencing or witnessing the trauma.
- Recurrent intrusions of reexperiencing the event via memories, nightmares, or dissociative reactions (e.g., flashbacks); intense distress at exposure to cues relating to the trauma; or physiological reactions to cues relating to the trauma.
- Active avoidance of triggering stimuli (e.g., memories, feelings, people, places, objects) associated with the trauma.
- At least two of the following negative cognitions/mood: dissociative amnesia, negative feelings of self/others/world, self-blame, negative emotions (e.g., fear, horror, anger, guilt), anhedonia, feelings of detachment/estrangement, inability to experience positive emotions.
- At least two of the following symptoms of $\uparrow$ arousal/reactivity: hypervigilance, exaggerated startle response, irritability/angry outbursts, impaired concentration, insomnia.
- Symptoms not caused by the direct effects of a substance or another medical condition.
- Symptoms result in significant impairment in social or occupational functioning.
- The presentation differs in children <7 years of age.

TABLE 5-4. **Posttraumatic Stress Disorder and Acute Stress Disorder**

POSTTRAUMATIC STRESS DISORDER	ACUTE STRESS DISORDER
Trauma occurred at any time in past	Trauma occurred <1 month ago
Symptoms last >1 month	Symptoms last <1 month

Epidemiology/Etiology

- Lifetime prevalence of PTSD: >8%
- Higher prevalence in women, most likely due to greater risk of exposure to traumatic events, particularly rape and other forms of interpersonal violence
- Exposure to prior trauma, especially during childhood, is a risk factor for developing PTSD.

Course/Prognosis

- PTSD usually begins within 3 months after the trauma.
- Symptoms of PTSD may have delayed expression.
- 50% of patients with PTSD have complete recovery within 3 months.
- Symptoms tend to diminish with older age.
- 80% of patients with PTSD have another mental disorder (e.g., MDD, bipolar disorder, anxiety disorder, substance use disorder).

Treatment

- **Pharmacological:**
  - First-line antidepressants: SSRIs (e.g., sertraline, citalopram) or SNRIs (e.g., venlafaxine)
  - Prazosin, α_1-receptor antagonist, targets **nightmares** and hypervigilance
  - May augment with atypical (second-generation) antipsychotics in severe cases.
- **Psychotherapy:**
  - Specialized forms of CBT (e.g., exposure therapy, cognitive processing therapy)
  - Supportive and psychodynamic therapy
  - Couples/family therapy

ADJUSTMENT DISORDERS

Adjustment disorders occur when behavioral or emotional symptoms develop after a stressful life event.

Diagnosis and DSM-5 Criteria

1. Development of emotional or behavioral symptoms within 3 months in response to an identifiable stressful life event. These symptoms produce either:
   - Marked distress in excess of what would be expected after such an event
   - Significant impairment in daily functioning
2. The symptoms are not those of normal bereavement.
3. Symptoms resolve within 6 months after stressor has terminated.
4. Stress-related disturbance does not meet criteria for another mental disorder.

Subtypes: Symptoms are coded based on a predominance of either depressed mood, anxiety, mixed anxiety and depression, disturbance of conduct (such as aggression), or mixed disturbance of emotions and conduct.

Epidemiology

- Adjustment disorders are very common (5–20% of patients in outpatient mental health clinics).
- They may occur at any age.

Etiology

Triggered by psychosocial factors.

Prognosis

May be chronic if the stressor is chronic or recurrent; symptoms (by definition) resolve within 6 months of cessation of stressor.

Treatment

- Supportive psychotherapy (most effective)
- Group therapy
- Occasionally pharmacotherapy is used to treat associated symptoms (insomnia, anxiety, or depression) in a time-limited fashion

CHAPTER 6

PERSONALITY DISORDERS

Definition   64
  DIAGNOSIS AND DSM-5 CRITERIA   64

Clusters   64
  ETIOLOGY   64
  TREATMENT   65

Cluster A   65
  PARANOID PERSONALITY DISORDER (PPD)   65
  SCHIZOID PERSONALITY DISORDER   66
  SCHIZOTYPAL PERSONALITY DISORDER   67

Cluster B   68
  ANTISOCIAL PERSONALITY DISORDER   69

BORDERLINE PERSONALITY DISORDER (BPD)   70
HISTRIONIC PERSONALITY DISORDER (HPD)   71
NARCISSISTIC PERSONALITY DISORDER (NPD)   72

Cluster C   73
  AVOIDANT PERSONALITY DISORDER   73
  DEPENDENT PERSONALITY DISORDER (DPD)   74
  OBSESSIVE-COMPULSIVE PERSONALITY DISORDER (OCPD) 75
  PERSONALITY CHANGE DUE TO ANOTHER MEDICAL
  CONDITION   76
  OTHER SPECIFIED PERSONALITY DISORDER   76
  UNSPECIFIED PERSONALITY DISORDER   76

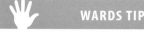

Definition

Personality is one's set of stable, predictable, emotional, and behavioral traits. Personality *disorders* involve enduring patterns of inner experience and behavior that deviate markedly from expectations of an individual's culture. They are pervasive, **maladaptive,** and cause significant impairment in social or occupational functioning. Patients with personality disorders often lack insight about their problems; their symptoms are either **ego-syntonic** or viewed as immutable. Patients with personality disorders are vulnerable to developing symptoms of other mental disorders during stress.

DIAGNOSIS AND DSM-5 CRITERIA

1. Enduring pattern of behavior/inner experience that deviates from the person's culture and is manifested in two or more of the following ways:
   - Cognition
   - Affect
   - Interpersonal functioning
   - Impulse control
2. The pattern:
   - Is **pervasive** and **inflexible** in a broad range of situations
   - Is **stable** and has an onset no later than adolescence or early adulthood
   - Leads to significant distress in functioning
   - Is not accounted for by another mental/medical illness or by use of a substance

The international prevalence of personality disorders is 6%. Personality disorders vary by gender. Many patients with personality disorders will meet the criteria for more than one disorder; they should be classified as having all of the disorders for which they qualify.

Clusters

Personality disorders are divided into three clusters:

- **Cluster A**—schizoid, schizotypal, and paranoid:
  - Patients seem eccentric, peculiar, or withdrawn.
  - Familial association with psychotic disorders.
- **Cluster B**—antisocial, borderline, histrionic, and narcissistic:
  - Patients seem emotional, dramatic, or inconsistent.
  - Familial association with mood disorders.
- **Cluster C**—avoidant, dependent, and obsessive-compulsive:
  - Patients seem anxious or fearful.
  - Familial association with anxiety disorders.

Other specified/unspecified personality disorder includes characteristics of a personality disorder that do not meet full criteria for any of the other personality disorders.

ETIOLOGY

- Biological, genetic, and psychosocial factors during childhood and adolescence contribute to the development of personality disorders.
- The prevalence of some personality disorders in monozygotic twins is several times higher than in dizygotic twins.

TREATMENT

- Personality disorders are generally very difficult to treat, especially since few patients are aware that they need help. The disorders tend to be chronic and lifelong.
- In general, pharmacologic treatment has limited usefulness (see individual exceptions below) except in treating comorbid mental conditions (e.g., major depressive disorder).
- Psychotherapy is usually the most helpful.

Cluster A

These patients are perceived as eccentric or odd by others and can have psychotic symptoms (Table 6-1).

PARANOID PERSONALITY DISORDER (PPD)

Patients with PPD have a pervasive distrust and suspiciousness of others and often interpret motives as malevolent. They tend to blame their own problems on others and seem angry and hostile. They are often characterized as being pathologically jealous, which leads them to think that their sexual partners or spouses are cheating on them.

Diagnosis and DSM-5 Criteria

- Diagnosis requires a general distrust of others, beginning by early adulthood and present in a variety of contexts.

TABLE 6-1. Cluster A Personality Disorders and Classic Clinical Examples

PERSONALITY DISORDER	CLINICAL EXAMPLE
Paranoid personality disorder	A 30-year-old man says his wife has been cheating on him because he does not have a good enough job to provide for her needs. He also claims that on his previous job, his boss laid him off because he did a better job than his boss. He has initiated several lawsuits. Refuses couples therapy because he believes the therapist will side with his wife. Believes neighbors are critical of him.
Schizoid personality disorder	A 45-year-old scientist works in the lab most of the day and has no friends, according to his coworkers. Has not been able to keep his job because of failure to collaborate with others. He expresses no desire to make friends and is content with his single life. He has no evidence of a thought disorder.
Schizotypal personality disorder	A 35-year-old man dresses in a wizard costume every weekend with friends as part of a live action role-playing community. He spends a great deal of time on his computers set up in his basement for video games and to "detect the presence of extraterrestrial communications in space." He has no auditory or visual hallucinations.

- At least four of the following must also be present:
  1. Suspicion (without evidence) that others are exploiting or deceiving him or her.
  2. Preoccupation with doubts of loyalty or trustworthiness of friends or acquaintances.
  3. Reluctance to confide in others.
  4. Interpretation of benign remarks as threatening or demeaning.
  5. Persistence of grudges.
  6. Perception of attacks on his or her character that is not apparent to others; quick to counterattack.
  7. Suspicions regarding fidelity of spouse or partner.

Epidemiology

- Prevalence: 2–4%.
- More commonly diagnosed in men than in women.
- Higher incidence in family members of schizophrenics.
- The disorder may be misdiagnosed in minority groups, immigrants, and deaf individuals.

Differential Diagnosis

- *Schizophrenia*: Unlike patients with schizophrenia, patients with PPD *do not have any fixed delusions and are not frankly psychotic*, although they may have transient psychosis under stressful situations.
- *Social disenfranchisement and social isolation*: Without a social support system, persons can react with suspicion to others. The differential in favor of the PPD can be assisted by the assessment of others in close contact with the person, who may identify what they consider as excess suspicion, etc.

Course and Prognosis

- The disorder usually has a chronic course, causing lifelong marital and job-related problems.

Treatment

- Psychotherapy is the treatment of choice.
- Group psychotherapy should be avoided due to mistrust and misinterpretation of others' statements.
- Patients may also benefit from a short course of antipsychotics for transient psychosis.

KEY FACT

Unlike with avoidant personality disorder, patients with schizoid personality disorder *prefer* to be alone.

SCHIZOID PERSONALITY DISORDER

Patients with schizoid personality disorder have a lifelong pattern of social withdrawal. They are often perceived as eccentric and reclusive. They are quiet and unsociable and have a constricted affect. They have *no desire for close relationships* and prefer to be alone.

Diagnosis and DSM-5 Criteria

- A pattern of voluntary social withdrawal and restricted range of emotional expression, beginning by early adulthood and present in a variety of contexts.
- Four or more of the following must also be present:
  1. Neither enjoying nor desiring close relationships (including family)
  2. Generally choosing solitary activities
  3. Little (if any) interest in sexual activity with another person
  4. Taking pleasure in few activities (if any)

5. Few close friends or confidants (if any)
6. Indifference to praise or criticism
7. Emotional coldness, detachment, or flattened affect

Epidemiology

- Prevalence: 3–5%.
- Diagnosed more often in men than women.
- May be ↑ prevalence of schizoid personality disorder in relatives of individuals with schizophrenia.

Differential Diagnosis

- *Schizophrenia*: Unlike patients with schizophrenia, patients with schizoid personality disorder do not have any fixed delusions or hallucinations.
- *Schizotypal personality disorder*: Patients with schizoid personality disorder do not have the same eccentric behavior or magical thinking seen in patients with schizotypal personality disorder. Schizotypal patients are more similar to schizophrenic patients in terms of odd perception, thought, and behavior.

Course

Usually chronic course.

Treatment

- Lack insight for individual psychotherapy, and may find group therapy threatening; may benefit from day programs or drop-in centers.
- Antidepressants if comorbid major depression is diagnosed.

SCHIZOTYPAL PERSONALITY DISORDER

Patients with schizotypal personality disorder have a pervasive pattern of eccentric behavior and peculiar thought patterns. They are often perceived as strange and odd. The disorder was developed out of the observation that certain family traits predominate in first-degree relatives of those with schizophrenia.

Diagnosis and DSM-5 Criteria

- A pattern of social deficits marked by eccentric behavior, cognitive or perceptual distortions, and discomfort with close relationships, beginning by early adulthood and present in a variety of contexts.
- Five or more of the following must be present:
  1. Ideas of reference (excluding delusions of reference)
  2. Odd beliefs or magical thinking, inconsistent with cultural norms
  3. Unusual perceptual experiences (such as bodily illusions)
  4. Suspiciousness
  5. Inappropriate or restricted affect
  6. Odd or eccentric appearance or behavior
  7. Few close friends or confidants
  8. Odd thinking or speech (vague, stereotyped, etc.)
  9. Excessive social anxiety
- Magical thinking may include:
  - Belief in clairvoyance or telepathy
  - Bizarre fantasies or preoccupations
  - Belief in superstitions
- Odd behaviors may include involvement in cults or strange religious practices.

Epidemiology

Prevalence: 4–5%.

Differential Diagnosis

- *Schizophrenia*: Unlike patients with schizophrenia, patients with schizotypal personality disorder are not frankly psychotic (though they can become transiently so under stress), nor do they have fixed delusions.
- *Schizoid personality disorder*: Patients with schizoid personality disorder do not have the same eccentric behavior seen in patients with schizotypal personality disorder.

Course

- Course is chronic, with small minority developing schizophrenia.
- Premorbid personality type for a patient with schizophrenia.

Treatment

- Psychotherapy is the treatment of choice to help develop social skills training.
- Short course of low-dose antipsychotics if necessary (for transient psychosis). Antipsychotics may help decrease social anxiety and suspicion in interpersonal relationships.

Cluster B

Includes antisocial, borderline, histrionic, and narcissistic personality disorders. These patients are often emotional, impulsive, and dramatic (Table 6-2).

TABLE 6-2.   Cluster B Personality Disorders and Classic Clinical Examples

PERSONALITY DISORDER	CLINICAL EXAMPLE
Antisocial personality disorder	A 30-year-old unemployed man has been accused of killing three senior citizens after robbing them. He is surprisingly charming in the interview. In his adolescence, he was arrested several times for stealing cars and assaulting other kids.
Borderline personality disorder	A 23-year-old medical student attempted to cut her wrist because things did not work out with a man she had been dating over the past 3 weeks. She states that guys are jerks and "not worth her time." She often feels that she is "alone in this world."
Histrionic personality disorder	A 33-year-old scantily clad woman comes to your office complaining that her fever feels like "she is burning in hell." She vividly describes how the fever has affected her work as a teacher.
Narcissistic personality disorder	A 48-year-old company CEO is rushed to the ED after an automobile accident. He does not let the residents operate on him and requests the Chief of trauma surgery because he is "vital to the company." He makes several business phone calls in the ED to stay on "top of his game."

Mr. Harris is a 35-year-old man with no prior psychiatric history who was arrested for assaulting his pregnant girlfriend. While in jail, he reports feeling depressed, and you are called in for a psychiatric evaluation. Mr. Harris is cooperative during the evaluation and presents as friendly and likeable. He reports that he is innocent of his charges and expresses feeling sad and tearful since his incarceration 2 days ago. He requests that you transfer him to the mental health unit at the correctional facility. However, you perform a thorough evaluation, and you do not find symptoms suggestive of a mood or psychotic disorder. When asked if he has been incarcerated before, he reports a history of multiple arrests and convictions for robbery and gun possession. He reports that he is unemployed because he has been "in and out of jail" during the past 5 years. He provides explanations for his limited involvement in these past crimes and does not appear remorseful.

Mr. Harris reveals a pattern of repeated fights since childhood and says that he quit school while in the ninth grade after being suspended for smoking pot on school grounds. Mr. Harris reports that throughout his childhood he bullied others, and laughs when recounting an episode during which he threw his cat against the wall to see it bounce back. He denies any family history of psychiatric illnesses, but reports that his father is currently incarcerated for drug trafficking.

What is his diagnosis?

Mr. Harris's diagnosis is antisocial personality disorder. His history shows a pervasive pattern of disregard for and violation of the rights of others since age 15, and there is evidence of conduct disorder with onset before age 15 years. Remember that, although it is common, not all criminals have antisocial personality disorder.

What are some associated findings?

Antisocial personality disorder is more prevalent in males, is associated with low socioeconomic background, and has a genetic predisposition. It has been found that the children of parents with antisocial personality disorder have an ↑ risk for this disorder, somatic symptom disorder, and substance use disorders.

ANTISOCIAL PERSONALITY DISORDER

A 26-year-old man has a history of multiple criminal arrests and is the son of two alcoholic parents. His brother recalls him setting their pet dog on fire as a kid. *Think: antisocial personality disorder.*

Antisocial personality disorder is a disorder in which a person violates the rights of others without showing guilt. Men, especially those with alcoholic parents, are more likely than women to have this condition.

Patients diagnosed with antisocial personality disorder are exploitive of others and break rules to meet their own needs. They lack empathy, compassion, and remorse for their actions. They are impulsive, deceitful, and often violate the law. They are frequently skilled at reading social cues and can appear charming and normal to others who meet them for the first time and do not know their history.

Diagnosis and DSM-5 Criteria

- Pattern of disregard for and violation of the rights of others since age 15.
- Patients must be **at least 18 years old** for this diagnosis; history of behavior as a child/adolescent must be consistent with **conduct disorder** (see chapter on Psychiatric Disorders in Children).
- Three or more of the following should be present:
  1. Failure to conform to social norms by committing unlawful acts
  2. Deceitfulness/repeated lying/manipulating others for personal gain
  3. Impulsivity/failure to plan ahead
  4. Irritability and aggressiveness/repeated fights or assaults
  5. Recklessness and disregard for safety of self or others
  6. Irresponsibility/failure to sustain work or honor financial obligations
  7. Lack of remorse for actions

Epidemiology

- Prevalence: 3% in men and 1% in women.
- There is a higher incidence in poor urban areas and in prisoners but no racial difference.
- Genetic component: ↑ risk among first-degree relatives.

Differential Diagnosis

Drug abuse: It is necessary to ascertain which came first. Patients who began abusing drugs before their antisocial behavior started may have behavior attributable to the effects of their addiction.

Course

- Usually has a chronic course, but some improvement of symptoms may occur as the patient ages.
- Many patients have multiple somatic complaints, and coexistence of substance use disorders and/or major depression is common.
- There is ↑ morbidity from substance use, trauma, suicide, or homicide.

Treatment

- Psychotherapy is generally ineffective.
- Pharmacotherapy may be used to treat symptoms of anxiety or depression, but use caution due to high addictive potential of these patients.

BORDERLINE PERSONALITY DISORDER (BPD)

Patients with BPD have unstable moods, behaviors, and interpersonal relationships. They fear abandonment and have poorly formed identity. Relationships begin with intense attachments and end with the slightest conflict. Aggression is common. They are impulsive and may have a history of repeated suicide attempts/gestures or episodes of self-mutilation. They have higher rates of childhood physical, emotional, and sexual abuse than the general population.

WARDS TIP

Symptoms of antisocial personality disorder—
CONDUCT
Capriciousness
Oppressive
Deceitful
Unlawful
Carefree
Temper

KEY FACT

Antisocial personality disorder begins in childhood as conduct disorder. Patient may have a history of being abused (physically or sexually) as a child or a history of hurting animals or starting fires. It is often associated with violations of the law.

Diagnosis and DSM-5 Criteria

- Pervasive pattern of impulsivity and unstable relationships, affects, self-image, and behaviors, present by early adulthood and in a variety of contexts.
- At least five of the following must be present:
  1. Frantic efforts to avoid real or imagined abandonment
  2. Unstable, intense interpersonal relationships (e.g., extreme love–hate relationships)
  3. Unstable self-image
  4. Impulsivity in at least two potentially harmful ways (spending, sexual activity, substance use, binge eating, etc.)
  5. Recurrent suicidal threats or attempts or self-mutilation
  6. Unstable mood/affect
  7. Chronic feelings of emptiness
  8. Difficulty controlling anger
  9. Transient, stress-related paranoid ideation or dissociative symptoms

Epidemiology

- Prevalence: Up to 6%.
- Diagnosed three times more often in women than men.
- Suicide rate: 10%.

Differential Diagnosis

- *Schizophrenia:* Unlike patients with schizophrenia, patients with BPD do not have frank psychosis (may have transient psychosis, however, if they decompensate under stress or substances of abuse).
- *Bipolar II:* Mood swings experienced in BPD are rapid, brief, moment-to-moment reactions to perceived environmental or psychological triggers.

Course

- Variable, but many develop stability in middle age.
- High incidence of coexisting major depression and/or substance use disorders.
- ↑ risk of suicide.

Treatment

- Psychotherapy (Dialectical Behavior Therapy, DBT) is the treatment of choice—includes cognitive-behavioral therapy, mindfulness skills, and group therapy.
- Pharmacotherapy to treat psychotic or depressive symptoms may be helpful.

HISTRIONIC PERSONALITY DISORDER (HPD)

Patients with HPD exhibit attention-seeking behavior and excessive emotionality. They are dramatic, flamboyant, and extroverted, but are unable to form long-lasting, meaningful relationships. They are often sexually inappropriate and provocative.

Diagnosis and DSM-5 Criteria

- Pattern of excessive emotionality and attention seeking, present by early adulthood and in a variety of contexts.
- At least five of the following must be present:
  1. Uncomfortable when not the center of attention
  2. Inappropriately seductive or provocative behavior

WARDS TIP

Symptoms of borderline personality disorder—
IMPULSIVE
Impulsive
Moody
Paranoid under stress
Unstable self-image
Labile, intense relationships
Suicidal
Inappropriate anger
Vulnerable to abandonment
Emptiness

WARDS TIP

Borderline patients commonly use the defense mechanism of *splitting*—they view others and themselves as all good or all bad. (Clinical example: "You are the only doctor who has ever helped me. Every doctor I met before you was horrible.")

WARDS TIP

Pharmacotherapy has been shown to be more useful in BPD than in any other personality disorder.

WARDS TIP

The name *borderline* comes from the patient's being on the borderline of neurosis and psychosis.

3. Rapidly shifting but shallow expression of emotion
4. Uses physical appearance to draw attention to self
5. Speech that is impressionistic and lacking in detail
6. Theatrical and exaggerated expression of emotion
7. Easily influenced by others or situation
8. Perceives relationships as more intimate than they actually are

Epidemiology

- Prevalence: 2%.
- Women are more likely to have HPD than men.

Differential Diagnosis

Borderline personality disorder: Patients with BPD are more likely to suffer from depression, brief psychotic episodes, and to attempt suicide. HPD patients are generally more functional.

Course

Usually chronic, with some improvement of symptoms with age.

Treatment

- Psychotherapy (e.g., supportive, problem-solving, interpersonal, group) is the treatment of choice.
- Pharmacotherapy to treat associated depressive or anxious symptoms as necessary.

> **WARDS TIP**
>
> Histrionic patients often use the defense mechanism of *regression*—they revert to childlike behaviors.

NARCISSISTIC PERSONALITY DISORDER (NPD)

Patients with NPD have a sense of superiority, a need for admiration, and a lack of empathy. They consider themselves "special" and will exploit others for their own gain. Despite their grandiosity, however, these patients often have fragile self-esteem.

Diagnosis and DSM-5 Criteria

- Pattern of grandiosity, need for admiration, and lack of empathy beginning by early adulthood and present in a variety of contexts.
- Five or more of the following must be present:
    1. Exaggerated sense of self-importance
    2. Preoccupation with fantasies of unlimited money, success, brilliance, etc.
    3. Believes that he or she is "special" or unique and can associate only with other high-status individuals
    4. Requires excessive admiration
    5. Has sense of entitlement
    6. Takes advantage of others for self-gain
    7. Lacks empathy
    8. Envious of others or believes others are envious of him or her
    9. Arrogant or haughty

Epidemiology

Prevalence: Up to 6%.

Differential Diagnosis

Antisocial personality disorder: Both types of patients exploit others, but NPD patients want status and recognition, while antisocial patients want material gain or simply the subjugation of others. Narcissistic patients become depressed when they don't get the recognition they think they deserve.

Course

Usually has a chronic course; higher incidence of depression and midlife crises since these patients put such a high value on youth and power.

Treatment

- Psychotherapy is the treatment of choice.
- Antidepressants may be used if a comorbid mood disorder is diagnosed.

Cluster C

Includes avoidant, dependent, and obsessive-compulsive personality disorders. These patients appear anxious and fearful (Table 6-3).

AVOIDANT PERSONALITY DISORDER

Patients with avoidant personality disorder have a pervasive pattern of social inhibition and an intense fear of rejection. They will avoid situations in which they may be rejected. Their fear of rejection is so overwhelming that it affects all aspects of their lives. They avoid social interactions and seek jobs in which there is little interpersonal contact. These patients *desire* companionship but are extremely shy and easily injured.

WARDS TIP

Narcissism is characterized by an inflated sense of entitlement. People with narcissistic personality are often "fishing for compliments" and become irritated and anxious when they are not treated as important.

KEY FACT

Avoidant personality disorder has large overlap with social anxiety disorder (social phobia); may be same syndrome/spectrum.

TABLE 6-3.   Cluster C Personality Disorders and Classic Clinical Examples

PERSONALITY DISORDER	CLINICAL EXAMPLE
Avoidant personality disorder	A 30-year-old postal worker rarely goes out with her coworkers and often makes excuses when they ask her to join them because she is afraid they will not like her. She wishes to go out and meet new people but, according to her, she is too "shy."
Dependent personality disorder	A 40-year-old man who lives with his parents has trouble deciding how to get his car fixed. He calls his father at work several times to ask very trivial things. He has been unemployed over the past 3 years.
Obsessive-compulsive personality disorder	A 40-year-old secretary has been recently fired because of her inability to prepare some work projects in time. According to her, they were not in the right format and she had to revise them six times, which led to the delay. This has happened before but she feels that she is not given enough time.

Diagnosis and DSM-5 Criteria

- A pattern of social inhibition, hypersensitivity, and feelings of inadequacy since early adulthood.
- At least four of the following must be present:
  1. Avoids occupation that involves interpersonal contact due to a fear of criticism and rejection
  2. Unwilling to interact unless certain of being liked
  3. Cautious of interpersonal relationships
  4. Preoccupied with being criticized or rejected in social situations
  5. Inhibited in new social situations because he or she feels inadequate
  6. Believes he or she is socially inept and inferior
  7. Reluctant to engage in new activities for fear of embarrassment

Epidemiology

- Prevalence: 2.4%.
- Equally frequent in males and females.

Differential Diagnosis

- *Schizoid personality disorder:* Patients with avoidant personality disorder desire companionship but are extremely shy, whereas patients with schizoid personality disorder have little or no desire for companionship.
- *Social anxiety disorder (social phobia):* See chapter on Anxiety Disorders. Both involve fear and avoidance of social situations. If the symptoms are an integral part of the patient's personality and have been evident since before adulthood, personality disorder is the more likely diagnosis. Social anxiety disorder involves a fear of *embarrassment* in a particular setting (speaking in public, urinating in public, etc.), whereas avoidant personality disorder is an overall fear of *rejection* and a sense of inadequacy. However, a patient can have both disorders concurrently and should carry both diagnoses if criteria for each are met.
- *Dependent personality disorder:* Avoidant personality disorder patients cling to relationships, similar to dependent personality disorder patients; however, avoidant patients are slow to get involved, whereas dependent patients actively and aggressively seek relationships.

Course

- Course is usually chronic, although may remit with age.
- Particularly difficult during adolescence, when attractiveness and socialization are important.
- ↑ incidence of associated anxiety and depressive disorders.
- If support system fails, patient is left very susceptible to depression, anxiety, and anger.

Treatment

- Psychotherapy, including assertiveness and social skills training, is most effective.
- Group therapy may also be beneficial.
- Selective serotonin reuptake inhibitors (SSRIs) may be prescribed for comorbid social anxiety disorder or major depression.

DEPENDENT PERSONALITY DISORDER (DPD)

Patients with DPD have poor self-confidence and fear of separation. They have an excessive need to be taken care of and allow others to make decisions for them. They feel helpless when left alone.

Diagnosis and DSM-5 Criteria

- A pattern of excessive need to be taken care of that leads to submissive and clinging behavior.
- At least five of the following must be present:
  1. Difficulty making everyday decisions without reassurance from others
  2. Needs others to assume responsibilities for most areas of his or her life
  3. Difficulty expressing disagreement because of fear of loss of approval
  4. Difficulty initiating projects because of lack of self-confidence
  5. Goes to excessive lengths to obtain support from others
  6. Feels helpless when alone
  7. Urgently seeks another relationship when one ends
  8. Preoccupied with fears of being left to take care of self

Epidemiology

- Prevalence: Approximately <1%.
- Women are more likely to be diagnosed with DPD than men.

Differential Diagnosis

- *Avoidant personality disorder:* See discussion above.
- *Borderline and histrionic personality disorders:* Patients with DPD usually have a long-lasting relationship with one person on whom they are dependent. Patients with borderline and histrionic personality disorders are often dependent on other people, but they are unable to maintain a long-lasting relationship.

Course

- Usually has a chronic course.
- Patients are prone to depression, particularly after loss of person on whom they are dependent.
- Difficulties with employment since they cannot act independently or without close supervision.

Treatment

- Psychotherapy, particularly cognitive-behavioral, assertiveness, and social skills training, is the treatment of choice.
- Pharmacotherapy may be used to treat associated symptoms of anxiety or depression.

OBSESSIVE-COMPULSIVE PERSONALITY DISORDER (OCPD)

Patients with OCPD have a pervasive pattern of perfectionism, inflexibility, and orderliness. They become so preoccupied with unimportant details that they are often unable to complete simple tasks in a timely fashion. They appear stiff, serious, and formal, with constricted affect. They are often successful professionally but have poor interpersonal skills.

Diagnosis and DSM-5 Criteria

- Pattern of preoccupation with orderliness, control, and perfectionism at the expense of efficiency and flexibility, present by early adulthood and in a variety of contexts.
- At least four of the following must be present:
  1. Preoccupation with details, rules, lists, and organization such that the major point of the activity is lost
  2. Perfectionism that is detrimental to completion of task

WARDS TIP

Symptoms of dependent personality disorder—
OBEDIENT
Obsessive about approval
Bound by other's decisions
Enterprises are rarely initiated due to their lack of self-confidence
Difficult to make own decisions
Invalid feelings while alone
Engrossed with fears of self-reliance
Needs to be in a relationship
Tentative about decisions

WARDS TIP

Many people with debilitating illnesses can develop dependent traits. However, to be diagnosed with DPD, the features must manifest in early adulthood.

3.   Excessive devotion to work
4.   Excessive conscientiousness and scrupulousness about morals and ethics
5.   Will not delegate tasks
6.   Unable to discard worthless objects
7.   Miserly spending style
8.   Rigid and stubborn

Epidemiology

- Prevalence: 1–2%.
- Men are two times more likely to have OCPD than women.

Differential Diagnosis

- *Obsessive-compulsive disorder (OCD)*: Patients with OCPD do not have the recurrent obsessions or compulsions that are present in OCD. In addition, the symptoms of OCPD are **ego-syntonic** rather than ego-dystonic (as in OCD); OCD patients are aware that they have a problem and wish that their thoughts and behaviors would go away.
- *Narcissistic personality disorder*: Both personalities involve assertiveness and achievement, but NPD patients are motivated by status, whereas OCPD patients are motivated by the work itself.

Course

- Unpredictable course.
- Some patients can have comorbid OCD (most do not).

> **KEY FACT**
>
> SSRIs often ↓ the intrusive thoughts associated with OCD.

Treatment

- Psychotherapy is the treatment of choice. Cognitive-behavior therapy may be particularly useful.
- Pharmacotherapy may be used to treat associated symptoms as necessary.

> **KEY FACT**
>
> As the name suggests, OCD is characterized by obsessions and compulsions. The obsession is the anxiety-producing thought aspect, while the compulsion is the behavioral aspect.

PERSONALITY CHANGE DUE TO ANOTHER MEDICAL CONDITION

This refers to a persistent personality change from a previous pattern due to the direct pathophysiological result of a medical condition (e.g., head trauma, strokes, epilepsy, central nervous system infections, or neoplasms). Subtypes include labile, disinhibited, aggressive, apathetic, or paranoid.

OTHER SPECIFIED PERSONALITY DISORDER

This diagnosis is reserved for a personality disorder that does not meet the full criteria for any of the disorders, but where the clinician *chooses* to communicate the specific reason that the presentation does not meet the criteria for any specific personality disorder (e.g., "mixed personality disorder").

UNSPECIFIED PERSONALITY DISORDER

This diagnosis is used for a personality disorder that does not meet the full criteria for any of the disorders, but where the clinician chooses *not* to specify the reason that the criteria are not met for any specific personality disorder (e.g., not enough information to make a more specific diagnosis).

NOTES

CHAPTER 7

SUBSTANCE-RELATED AND ADDICTIVE DISORDERS

Substance Use Disorders	80
DIAGNOSIS AND DSM-5 CRITERIA	80
EPIDEMIOLOGY	80
PSYCHIATRIC SYMPTOMS	80
ACUTE INTOXICATION AND WITHDRAWAL	80
DETECTION OF SUBSTANCE USE	81
TREATMENT OF SUBSTANCE USE DISORDERS	81
Alcohol (EtOH)	81
INTOXICATION	82
WITHDRAWAL	83
ALCOHOL USE DISORDER	85
Cocaine	87
INTOXICATION	87
COCAINE USE DISORDER	87
WITHDRAWAL	87
Amphetamines	87
INTOXICATION	88
Phencyclidine (PCP)	88
INTOXICATION	88
WITHDRAWAL	89
Sedative-Hypnotics	89
INTOXICATION	89
WITHDRAWAL	89
Opioids	90
INTOXICATION	90
OPIATE USE DISORDER	90
WITHDRAWAL	90
Hallucinogens	91
INTOXICATION	92
WITHDRAWAL	92
Marijuana	92
INTOXICATION	92
WITHDRAWAL	92
Inhalants	93
INTOXICATION	93
WITHDRAWAL	93
Caffeine	93
OVERDOSE	93
WITHDRAWAL	94
Nicotine	94
TREATMENT OF NICOTINE DEPENDENCE	94
Gambling Disorder	94
DIAGNOSIS AND DSM-5 CRITERIA	94
EPIDEMIOLOGY/ETIOLOGY	95
TREATMENT	95

Substance Use Disorders

DIAGNOSIS AND DSM-5 CRITERIA

Cognitive, behavioral, and physiological symptoms indicating continuous use of a substance despite significant substance-related problems.

Substance use disorder characterized by a problematic pattern of substance use → impairment or distress manifested by at least two of the following within a 12-month period (note that these criteria are the same regardlnes of the substance):

1. Using substance more than originally intended
2. Persistent desire or unsuccessful efforts to cut down on use
3. Significant time spent in obtaining, using, or recovering from substance
4. Craving to use substance
5. Failure to fulfill obligations at work, school, or home
6. Continued use despite social or interpersonal problems due to the substance use
7. ↓ social, occupational, or recreational activities because of substance use
8. Use in dangerous situations (e.g., driving a car)
9. Continued use despite subsequent physical or psychological problem (e.g., drinking alcohol despite worsening liver problems)
10. Tolerance (see definition below)
11. Withdrawal (see definition below)

EPIDEMIOLOGY

- One-year prevalence of any substance use disorder in the United States is approximately 8%.
- More common in men than women.
- Alcohol and nicotine are the most commonly used substances.

PSYCHIATRIC SYMPTOMS

- Mood symptoms are common among persons with substance use disorders.
- Psychotic symptoms may occur with some substances.
- Personality disorders and psychiatric comorbidities (e.g., major depression, anxiety disorders) are common among persons with substance use disorders.
- It is often challenging to decide whether psychiatric symptoms are primary or substance-induced.
- **Withdrawal:** The development of a substance-specific syndrome due to the cessation (or reduction) of substance use that has been heavy and prolonged.
- **Tolerance:** The need for ↑ amounts of the substance to achieve the desired effect *or* diminished effect if using the same amount of the substance.

ACUTE INTOXICATION AND WITHDRAWAL

Both the intoxicated and withdrawing patient can present difficulties in diagnosis and treatment. Since it is common for persons to abuse several substances at once, the clinical presentation is often confusing, and signs/symptoms may be atypical. Always be on the lookout for multiple substance use.

WARDS TIP

It is possible to have a substance use disorder without having physiological dependence (i.e., without having withdrawal or tolerance).

WARDS TIP

Substance-induced mood symptoms improve during abstinence, whereas *primary* mood symptoms persist.

KEY FACT

Withdrawal symptoms of a drug are usually opposite of its intoxication effects. For example, alcohol is sedating, but alcohol withdrawal can → brain excitation and seizures.

TABLE 7-1. **Direct Testing for Substance Use**

Alcohol	■ Stays in system for only a few hours.
	■ Breathalyzer test, commonly used by police enforcement.
	■ Blood/urine testing more accurate.
Cocaine	■ Urine drug screen positive for 2–4 days.
Amphetamines	■ Urine drug screen positive for 1–3 days.
	■ Most assays are not of adequate sensitivity or specificity.
Phencyclidine (PCP)	■ Urine drug screen positive for 4–7 days.
	■ Creatine phosphokinase (CPK) and aspartate aminotransferase (AST) are often elevated.
Sedative-hypnotics	In urine and blood for variable amounts of time.
	Barbiturates:
	■ Short-acting (pentobarbital): 24 hours
	■ Long-acting (phenobarbital): 3 weeks
	Benzodiazepines:
	■ Short-acting (e.g., lorazepam): up to 5 days
	■ Long-acting (diazepam): up to 30 days
Opioids	■ Urine drug test remains positive for 1–3 days, depending on opioid used.
	■ Methadone and oxycodone will come up negative on a general screen (order a separate panel).
Marijuana	Urine detection:
	■ After a single use, about 3 days. In heavy users, up to 4 weeks (THC is released from adipose stores).

KEY FACT

Pregnant women should not drink alcohol as it can → fetal alcohol syndrome in the newborn, which is one of the leading causes of intellectual disability (mental retardation) in the United States.

DETECTION OF SUBSTANCE USE

See Table 7-1.

TREATMENT OF SUBSTANCE USE DISORDERS

- Behavioral counseling should be part of every substance use disorder treatment.
- Psychosocial treatments are effective and include motivational intervention (MI), cognitive-behavioral therapy (CBT), contingency management, and individual and group therapy.
- Twelve-step groups such as Alcoholics Anonymous (AA) and Narcotics Anonymous (NA) should also be encouraged as part of the treatment.
- Pharmacotherapy is available for some drugs of abuse, and will be discussed later in this chapter as relevant to a particular substance.

Alcohol (EtOH)

- Alcohol activates gamma-aminobutyric acid (GABA), dopamine, and serotonin receptors in the central nervous system (CNS), and inhibits glutamate receptor activity and voltage-gated calcium channels. GABA receptors are inhibitory, and glutamate receptors are excitatory. Thus, alcohol is a potent CNS depressant.

- Lifetime prevalence of alcohol use disorder in the United States is 5% of women and 12% of men.
- Alcohol is metabolized in the following manner:
  1. Alcohol → acetaldehyde (enzyme: *alcohol dehydrogenase*).
  2. Acetaldehyde → acetic acid (enzyme: *aldehyde dehydrogenase*).

There is upregulation of these enzymes in heavy drinkers. Secondary to a gene variant, Asians often have less aldehyde dehydrogenase, resulting in flushing and nausea, and likely reducing their risk of alcohol use disorder.

INTOXICATION

Clinical Presentation

- The absorption and elimination rates of alcohol are variable and depend on many factors, including age, sex, body weight, chronic nature of use, duration of consumption, food in the stomach, and the state of nutrition and liver health.
- In addition to the above factors, the effects of EtOH also depend on the blood alcohol level (BAL). Serum EtOH level or an expired air breathalyzer can determine the extent of intoxication. As shown in Table 7-2, the effects/BAL may be ↓ if high tolerance has been developed.

Treatment

- **Monitor:** Airway, breathing, circulation, glucose, electrolytes, acid–base status.
- Give **thiamine** (to prevent or treat Wernicke's encephalopathy) and folate.
- **Naloxone** may be necessary to reverse effects of co-ingested opioids.
- A computed tomographic (CT) scan of the head may be necessary to rule out subdural hematoma or other brain injury.
- The liver will eventually metabolize alcohol without any other interventions.
- Severely intoxicated patient may require mechanical ventilation with attention to acid–base balance, temperature, and electrolytes while he or she is recovering.
- Gastrointestinal evacuation (e.g., gastric lavage, induction of emesis, and charcoal) is not indicated in the treatment of EtOH overdose unless a significant amount of EtOH was ingested within the preceding 30–60 minutes.

TABLE 7-2. Clinical Presentation of Alcohol Intoxication

EFFECTS	BAL
↓ fine motor control	20–50 mg/dL
Impaired judgment and coordination	50–100 mg/dL
Ataxic gait and poor balance	100–150 mg/dL
Lethargy, difficulty sitting upright, difficulty with memory, nausea/vomiting	150–250 mg/dL
Coma in the novice drinker	300 mg/dL
Respiratory depression, death possible	400 mg/dL

WITHDRAWAL

A 42-year-old man has routine surgery for a knee injury. After 72 hours in the hospital he becomes anxious, flushed, diaphoretic, hypertensive, and tachycardic. *What most likely can account for this patient's symptoms?* Alcohol withdrawal. *Treatment?* Benzodiazepine taper (chlordiazepoxide [Librium] or lorazepam [Ativan] are considered the drugs of choice). *What are you most concerned about?* Seizures, delirium, hypertension, and arrhythmias.

Chronic alcohol use has a depressant effect on the CNS, and cessation of use causes a compensatory hyperactivity. Alcohol withdrawal is *potentially lethal!*

Clinical Presentation

- Signs and symptoms of **alcohol withdrawal syndrome** include insomnia, anxiety, hand tremor, irritability, anorexia, nausea, vomiting, autonomic hyperactivity (diaphoresis, tachycardia, hypertension), psychomotor agitation, fever, seizures, hallucinations, and delirium (see Table 7-3).
- The earliest symptoms of EtOH withdrawal begin between 6 and 24 hours after the patient's last drink and depend on the duration and quantity of EtOH consumption.
- Generalized tonic-clonic seizures usually occur between 12 and 48 hours after cessation of drinking, with a peak around 12–24 hours.
- About a third of persons with seizures develop delirium tremens (DTs).
- Hypomagnesemia may predispose to seizures; thus, it should be corrected promptly.
- Seizures are treated with benzodiazepines. Long-term treatment with anticonvulsants is not recommended for alcohol withdrawal seizures.

Delirium Tremens (DTs)

- The most serious form of EtOH withdrawal.
- Usually begins 48–96 hours after the last drink but may occur later.
- While only 5% of patients who experience EtOH withdrawal develop DTs, there is a roughly 5% mortality rate (up to 35% if left untreated).
- Physical illness predisposes to the condition.
- Age >30 and prior DTs increase the risk.
- In addition to delirium, symptoms of DTs may include hallucinations (most commonly visual), agitation, gross tremor, autonomic instability, and fluctuating levels of psychomotor activity.
- It is a medical emergency and should be treated with adequate doses of benzodiazepines.

KEY FACT

Alcohol is the most commonly used intoxicating substance in the United States.

KEY FACT

Attempted suicide is associated with mental illness, young females, and alcohol use.

KEY FACT

Delirium tremens carries a 5% mortality rate but occurs in only 5% of patients that experience EtOH withdrawal.

TABLE 7-3. Alcohol Withdrawal Symptoms

EtOH withdrawal symptoms usually begin in 6–24 hours and last 2–7 days.
Mild: Irritability, tremor, insomnia.
Moderate: Diaphoresis, hypertension, tachycardia, fever, disorientation.
Severe: Tonic-clonic seizures, DTs, hallucinations.

KEY FACT

Confabulations, or inventing stories of events that never occurred, are often associated with Korsakoff's "psychosis," or alcohol-induced neurocognitive disorder. Patients are unaware that they are "making these up."

Treatment

- Benzodiazepines (chlordiazepoxide, diazepam, or lorazepam) should be given in sufficient doses to keep the patient calm and lightly sedated, then tapered down slowly. Carbamazepine or valproic acid can be used in mild withdrawal.
- Antipsychotics (be careful of lowering seizure threshold) and temporary restraints for severe agitation.
- Thiamine, folic acid, and a multivitamin to treat nutritional deficiencies ("banana bag").
- Electrolyte and fluid abnormalities must be corrected.
- Monitor withdrawal signs and symptoms with Clinical Institute Withdrawal Assessment (CIWA) scale.
- Careful attention must be given to the level of consciousness, and the possibility of trauma should be investigated.
- Check for signs of hepatic failure (e.g., ascites, jaundice, caput medusae, coagulopathy).

Mr. Smith is a 42-year-old divorced man who arrives to the ED requesting treatment for alcohol detoxification. He began drinking at the age of 17 and, although he initially drank only on the weekends, his alcohol use progressively increased to drinking half a pint of whiskey daily by the age of 35. At that time, he was referred to a 45-day inpatient alcohol abuse program after he arrived intoxicated at his workplace on several occasions, and after completion of the program, he was able to maintain sobriety for 7 years. However, 2 years ago he relapsed into alcohol use after he divorced and was laid off from work due to "the economy."

Mr. Smith is currently living with his older sister and states that his drinking is "out of control." He had a DUI recently and has a court date in 2 weeks. He has tried to quit alcohol on his own on several occasions. However, when he stops drinking he feels "shaky, sweaty, anxious, and irritable" and thus resumes his alcohol intake. He also reports a history of a seizure 10 years ago, after he abruptly discontinued his alcohol use during a few days.

Mr. Smith's last drink was about 8 hours prior to his arrival at the ED. During the last month he has been feeling sad, with low energy, difficulty falling and staying asleep, ↓ appetite, and difficulty concentrating. He denies suicidal ideation but has significant guilt over not being able to stop drinking. He denies a history of depression or anxiety, and has not received any other psychiatric treatment in the past.

Upon presentation to ER the patient's breathalyzer was 0.11, he did not have symptoms of intoxication, and his urine drug screen was negative. Vital signs were significant for blood pressure of 150/90 and pulse of 110 bpm. Complete blood count and electrolytes were within normal limits.

What is Mr. Smith's most likely diagnosis?

The patient has a diagnosis of alcohol use disorder. It is clear that he has exhibited symptoms of tolerance and withdrawal, has been using more alcohol than intended, and has made unsuccessful efforts to cut down. He also describes symptoms suggestive of a depressive disorder.

The fact that his depressive symptoms began while abusing alcohol warrants a diagnosis of alcohol-induced depressive disorder. However, major depressive disorder should be ruled out once he remits his alcohol use. If his depressive symptoms are indeed substance-induced, they will improve and resolve with continuing sobriety.

What would be the next step in management?

Given the Mr. Smith's heavy chronic alcohol use and history of complicated withdrawal (i.e., seizure), he should be admitted to an inpatient unit for close monitoring. Outpatient detoxification is not appropriate in this case. He will likely require a standing and PRN benzodiazepine (the particular benzodiazepine sometimes varies depending on hospital's protocol), and will be close monitoring for signs of withdrawal.

ALCOHOL USE DISORDER

- The **AUDIT-C** (Table 7-4) is used to screen for alcohol use disorder.
- Biochemical markers are useful in detecting recent prolonged drinking; ongoing monitoring of biomarkers can also help detect a relapse. Most commonly used biomarkers are BAL, liver function tests (LFTs—aspartate aminotransferase [AST], alanine aminotransferase [ALT]), gamma-glutamyl transpeptidase (GGT), and mean corpuscular volume (MCV).

Medications for Alcohol Use Disorder

First-line treatments:
- Naltrexone (Revia, IM-Vivitrol):
  - Opioid receptor blocker.
  - Works by ↓ desire/craving and "high" associated with alcohol.
  - Maybe greater benefit is seen in men with a family history of alcoholism.
  - In patients with physical opioid dependence, it will precipitate withdrawal.
- Acamprosate (Campral):
  - Thought to modulate glutamate transmission.
  - Should be started post-detoxification for relapse prevention in patients who have stopped drinking.
  - Major advantage is that it can be used in patients with liver disease.
  - Contraindicated in severe renal disease.

Second-line treatments:
- Disulfiram (Antabuse):
  - Blocks the enzyme aldehyde dehydrogenase in the liver and causes aversive reaction to alcohol (flushing, headache, nausea/vomiting, palpitations, shortness of breath).
  - Contraindicated in severe cardiac disease, pregnancy, psychosis.
  - Liver function should be monitored.
  - Best used in highly motivated patients, as medication adherence is an issue.
- Topiramate (Topamax):
  - Anticonvulsant that potentiates GABA and inhibits glutamate receptors.
  - Reduces cravings for alcohol and decreases alcohol use.

WARDS TIP

At-risk or heavy drinking for men is > 4 drinks per day or > 14 drinks per week. For women, it is > 3 drinks per day or > 7 drinks per week.

KEY FACT

AST:ALT ratio ≥ 2:1 and elevated GGT suggest excessive alcohol use.

KEY FACT

Alcohol can cause ↑ LFTs and macrocytosis (↑ MCV).

KEY FACT

Delirium tremens is a dangerous form of alcohol withdrawal involving mental status and neurological changes. Symptoms include disorientation; agitation; visual and tactile hallucinations; and ↑ respiratory rate, heart rate, and blood pressure. Treatment includes supportive care and benzodiazepines.

TABLE 7-4. AUDIT-C

QUESTION #1: HOW OFTEN DID YOU HAVE A DRINK CONTAINING ALCOHOL IN THE PAST YEAR?

▪ Never	(0 points)
▪ Monthly or less	(1 point)
▪ Two to four times a month	(2 points)
▪ Two to three times per week	(3 points)
▪ Four or more times a week	(4 points)

QUESTION #2: HOW MANY DRINKS DID YOU HAVE ON A TYPICAL DAY WHEN YOU WERE DRINKING IN THE PAST YEAR?

▪ 1 or 2	(0 points)
▪ 3 or 4	(1 point)
▪ 5 or 6	(2 points)
▪ 7 to 9	(3 points)
▪ 10 or more	(4 points)

QUESTION #3: HOW OFTEN DID YOU HAVE SIX OR MORE DRINKS ON ONE OCCASION IN THE PAST YEAR?

▪ Never	(0 points)
▪ Less than monthly	(1 point)
▪ Monthly	(2 points)
▪ Weekly	(3 points)
▪ Daily or almost daily	(4 points)

The AUDIT-C is scored on a scale of 0–12 (scores of 0 reflect no alcohol use). In men, a score of 4 or more is considered positive; in women, a score of 3 or more is considered positive.

WARDS TIP

All patients with altered mental status should be given thiamine *before* glucose, or Wernicke–Korsakoff syndrome may be precipitated. Thiamine is a coenzyme used in carbohydrate metabolism.

Long-Term Complications of Alcohol Intake

- **Wernicke's encephalopathy:**
  - Caused by thiamine (vitamin B_1) deficiency resulting from poor nutrition.
  - Acute and can be reversed with thiamine therapy.
  - Features: Ataxia (broad-based), confusion, ocular abnormalities (nystagmus, gaze palsies).
- If left untreated, Wernicke's encephalopathy may progress to **Korsakoff syndrome:**
  - Chronic amnestic syndrome.
  - Reversible in only about 20% of patients.
  - Features: Impaired recent memory, anterograde amnesia, compensatory confabulation (unconsciously making up answers when memory has failed).

Cocaine

Cocaine blocks the reuptake of dopamine, epinephrine, and norepinephrine from the synaptic cleft, causing a stimulant effect. Dopamine plays a role in the behavioral reinforcement ("reward") system of the brain.

INTOXICATION

- *General:* Euphoria, heightened self-esteem, ↑ or ↓ blood pressure, tachycardia or bradycardia, nausea, dilated pupils, weight loss, psychomotor agitation or depression, chills, and sweating.
- *Dangerous:* Respiratory depression, seizures, arrhythmias, hyperthermia, paranoia, and hallucinations (especially tactile). Since cocaine is an indirect sympathomimetic, intoxication mimics the fight-or-flight response.
- *Deadly:* Cocaine's vasoconstrictive effect may result in myocardial infarction (MI), intracranial hemorrhage, or stroke.

Management

- For mild-to-moderate agitation and anxiety: Reassurance of the patient and benzodiazepines.
- For severe agitation or psychosis: Antipsychotics (e.g., haloperidol).
- Symptomatic support (i.e., control hypertension, arrhythmias).
- Temperature of >102°F should be treated aggressively with ice bath, cooling blanket, and other supportive measures.

COCAINE USE DISORDER

Treatment of cocaine use disorder
- There is no FDA-approved pharmacotherapy for cocaine dependence.
- Off-label medications are sometimes used (disulfiram, modafinil, topiramate).
- Psychological interventions (contingency management, relapse prevention, NA, etc.) are efficacious and the mainstay of treatment.

WITHDRAWAL

- Abrupt abstinence is not life threatening.
- Produces post-intoxication depression ("crash"): Malaise, fatigue, hypersomnolence, depression, anhedonia, hunger, constricted pupils, vivid dreams, psychomotor agitation, or retardation. Occasionally, these patients can become suicidal.
- With mild-to-moderate cocaine use, withdrawal symptoms resolve within 72 hours; with heavy, chronic use, they may last for 1–2 weeks.
- Treatment is supportive, but severe psychiatric symptoms may warrant hospitalization.

Amphetamines

- Classic amphetamines:
  - Block reuptake and facilitate release of dopamine and norepinephrine from nerve endings, causing a stimulant effect.
  - *Examples:* Dextroamphetamine (Dexedrine), methylphenidate (Ritalin), methamphetamine (Desoxyn, "ice," "speed," "crystal meth," "crank").

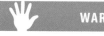

KEY FACT

Remember, the symptoms of amphetamine abuse are euphoria, dilated pupils, ↑ libido, tachycardia, perspiration, grinding teeth, chest pain.

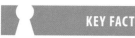

WARDS TIP

Chronic amphetamine use → accelerated tooth decay ("meth mouth").

WARDS TIP

Amphetamine use is associated with ↑ tolerance, but also can → seizures.

KEY FACT

Ketamine ("special K") can produce tachycardia, tachypnea, hallucinations, and amnesia.

KEY FACT

PCP intoxication symptoms—
RED DANES
Rage
Erythema (redness of skin)
Dilated pupils
Delusions
Amnesia
Nystagmus
Excitation
Skin dryness

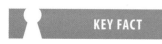

KEY FACT

Rotatory nystagmus is strongly suggestive for PCP intoxication.

- Methamphetamines are easily manufactured in home laboratories using over-the-counter medications (e.g., pseudoephedrine).
  - They are used medically in the treatment of narcolepsy, attention deficit/hyperactivity disorder (ADHD), and occasionally depressive disorders.
- Substituted ("designer," "club drugs") amphetamines:
  - Release dopamine, norepinephrine, and serotonin from nerve endings.
  - *Examples:* MDMA ("ecstasy"), MDEA ("eve").
  - These substances are associated with dance clubs and raves.
  - Have both stimulant and hallucinogenic properties.
  - Serotonin syndrome is possible if designer amphetamines are combined with selective serotonin reuptake inhibitors (SSRIs).

INTOXICATION

Clinical Presentation

- Amphetamine intoxication causes symptoms similar to those of cocaine (see above).
- MDMA and MDEA may induce sense of closeness to others.
- Overdose can → hyperthermia, dehydration (especially after a prolonged period of dancing in a club), rhabdomyolysis, and renal failure.
- Complications of their long half-life can cause ongoing psychosis, even during abstinence.
- Amphetamine withdrawal can → prolonged depression.

Treatment

Rehydrate, correct electrolyte balance, and treat hyperthermia.

Phencyclidine (PCP)

PCP, or "angel dust," is a dissociative, hallucinogenic drug that antagonizes N-methyl-D-aspartate (NMDA) glutamate receptors and activates dopaminergic neurons. It can have stimulant or CNS depressant effects, depending on the dose taken.

- PCP can be smoked as "wet" (sprinkled on cigarette) or as a "joint" (sprinkled on marijuana).
- Ketamine is similar to PCP, but is less potent. Ketamine is sometimes used as a "date rape" drug, as it is odorless and tasteless.

INTOXICATION

Clinical Presentation

- Effects include agitation, depersonalization, hallucinations, synesthesia (one sensory stimulation evokes another, such as hearing a sound producing a color), impaired judgment, memory impairment, assaultiveness, **nystagmus** (rotary, horizontal, or vertical), ataxia, dysarthria, hypertension, tachycardia, muscle rigidity, and high tolerance to pain.
- Overdose can cause seizures, delirium, coma, and even death.

Treatment

- Monitor vitals, temperature, and electrolytes, and minimize sensory stimulation.
- Use benzodiazepines (lorazepam) to treat agitation, anxiety, muscle spasms, and seizures.
- Use antipsychotics (haloperidol) to control severe agitation or psychotic symptoms.

WITHDRAWAL

No withdrawal syndrome, but "flashbacks" (recurrence of intoxication symptoms due to release of the drug from body lipid stores) may occur.

Sedative-Hypnotics

Agents in the sedative-hypnotics category include benzodiazepines, barbiturates, zolpidem, zaleplon, gamma-hydroxybutyrate (GHB), meprobamate, and others. These medications, especially benzodiazepines, are highly abused in the United States, as they are more readily available than other drugs such as cocaine or opioids.

- Benzodiazepines (BDZs):
  - Commonly used in the treatment of anxiety disorders.
  - Easily obtained via prescription from physician offices and emergency departments.
  - Potentiate the effects of GABA by modulating the receptor, thereby ↑ the frequency of chloride channel opening.
- Barbiturates:
  - Used in the treatment of epilepsy and as anesthetics.
  - Potentiate the effects of GABA by binding to the receptor and ↑ the duration of chloride channel opening.
  - At high doses, barbiturates act as direct GABA agonists, and therefore have a lower margin of safety relative to BDZs.
  - They are synergistic in combination with BDZs (as well as other CNS depressants such as alcohol); respiratory depression can occur as a complication.

INTOXICATION

Clinical Presentation

- Intoxication with sedatives produces drowsiness, confusion, hypotension, slurred speech, incoordination, ataxia, mood lability, impaired judgment, nystagmus, respiratory depression, and coma or death in overdose.
- Symptoms are synergistic when combined with EtOH or opioids/narcotics.
- Long-term sedative use may → dependence and may cause depressive symptoms.

Treatment

- Maintain airway, breathing, and circulation. Monitor vital signs.
- Activated charcoal and gastric lavage to prevent further gastrointestinal absorption (if drug was ingested in the prior 4–6 hours).
- For *barbiturates only*: Alkalinize urine with sodium bicarbonate to promote renal excretion.
- For *benzodiazepines only*: Flumazenil in overdose.
- Supportive care—improve respiratory status, control hypotension.

WITHDRAWAL

Abrupt abstinence after chronic use can be *life threatening*. While physiological dependence is more likely with short-acting agents, longer-acting agents can also cause dependence and withdrawal symptoms.

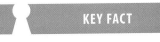

KEY FACT

Tactile and visual hallucinations are found in both cocaine and PCP intoxication.

KEY FACT

More than with other drugs, intoxication with PCP results in violence.

KEY FACT

Gamma-hydroxybutyrate (GHB) is a dose-specific CNS depressant that produces confusion, dizziness, drowsiness, memory loss, respiratory distress, and coma. It is commonly used as a date-rape drug.

KEY FACT

Barbiturate withdrawal can be deadly. Of all the kinds of drug withdrawals, withdrawal from barbiturates has the highest mortality rate.

WARDS TIP

Flumazenil is a very short-acting BDZ antagonist used for treating BDZ overdose. Use with caution when treating overdose, as it may precipitate seizures.

Clinical Presentation

Signs and symptoms of withdrawal are the same as these of EtOH withdrawal. Tonic-clonic seizures may occur and can be life threatening.

Treatment

- Benzodiazepine taper.
- Carbamazepine or valproic acid taper not as beneficial.

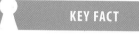

Opioids

- Opioid medications and drugs of abuse stimulate mu, kappa, and delta opiate receptors (normally stimulated by endogenous opiates), and are involved in analgesia, sedation, and dependence. Examples include heroin, oxycodone, codeine, dextromethorphan, morphine, methadone, and meperidine (Demerol).
- Opioids also have effects on the dopaminergic system, which mediates their addictive and rewarding properties.
- Prescription opioids (OxyContin [oxycodone], Vicodin [hydrocodone/acetaminophen], and Percocet [oxycodone/acetaminophen]), not heroin, are the most commonly used opioids.
- Behaviors such as losing medication, "doctor shopping," and running out of medication early should alert clinician of possible misuse.

INTOXICATION

Clinical Presentation

- Opioid intoxication causes drowsiness, nausea/vomiting, constipation, slurred speech, **constricted pupils**, seizures, and respiratory depression, which may progress to coma or death in overdose.
- Meperidine and monoamine oxidase inhibitors taken in combination may cause the **serotonin syndrome**: hyperthermia, confusion, hyper- or hypotension, and muscular rigidity.

Treatment

- Ensure adequate airway, breathing, and circulation.
- In overdose, administration of naloxone (opioid antagonist) will improve respiratory depression but may cause severe withdrawal in an opioid-dependent patient.
- Ventilatory support may be required.

OPIATE USE DISORDER

See Table 7-5 for treatment of opioid use disorder.

WITHDRAWAL

- While not life threatening, abstinence in the opioid-dependent individual leads to an unpleasant withdrawal syndrome characterized by dysphoria, insomnia, lacrimation, rhinorrhea, yawning, weakness, sweating, piloerection, nausea/vomiting, fever, dilated pupils, abdominal cramps, arthralgia, myalgia, hypertension, tachycardia, and craving.

KEY FACT

In general, withdrawal from drugs that are sedating (e.g., alcohol, barbiturates, benzodiazepines) is life threatening, while withdrawal from stimulants (e.g., cocaine, amphetamines) is not.

KEY FACT

The opioid dextromethorphan is a common ingredient in cough syrup.

KEY FACT

Infection secondary to needle sharing is a common cause of morbidity from street heroin usage.

KEY FACT

Opioid intoxication: nausea, vomiting, sedation, ↓ pain perception, ↓ gastrointestinal motility, pupil constriction, and respiratory depression (which *can be fatal*).

KEY FACT

Meperidine is the exception to opioids producing miosis. "Demerol Dilates pupils."

WARDS TIP

Classic triad of opioid overdose—
Rebels Admire Morphine
Respiratory depression
Altered mental status
Miosis

KEY FACT

Naloxone is the treatment of choice for opiate overdose.

TABLE 7-5. **Pharmacological Treatment of Opioid Use Disorder**

MEDICATION	MECHANISM	PROS	CONS
Methadone	Long-acting opioid receptor agonist	Administered once daily. Significantly reduces morbidity and mortality in opioid-dependent persons. "Gold standard" treatment in pregnant opioid-dependent women.	Restricted to federally licensed substance abuse treatment programs. Can cause QTc interval prolongation; thus, screening electrocardiogram is indicated, particularly for certain patients such as those with cardiac disease.
Buprenorphine	Partial opioid receptor agonist	Sublingual preparation that is safer than methadone, as its effects reach a plateau and make overdose unlikely. Comes as Suboxone, which contains buprenorphine and naloxone; more commonly used, as this preparation prevents intoxication from intravenous injection.	Available by prescription from office-based physicians.
Naltrexone	Competitive opioid antagonist, precipitates withdrawal if used within 7 days of heroin use	Either daily orally or monthly depot injection. It is a good choice for highly motivated patients such as health care professionals.	Compliance is an issue.

- Treatment includes:
  - Moderate symptoms: Symptomatic treatment with clonidine (for autonomic signs and symptoms of withdrawal), nonsteroidal anti-inflammatory drugs (NSAIDs) for pain, dicyclomine for abdominal cramps, etc.
  - Severe symptoms: Detox with buprenorphine or methadone.
  - Monitor degree of withdrawal with COWS (Clinical Opioid Withdrawal Scale), which uses objective measures (i.e., pulse, pupil size, tremor) to assess withdrawal severity.

Hallucinogens

Hallucinogenic drugs of abuse include psilocybin (mushrooms), mescaline (peyote cactus), and lysergic acid diethylamide (LSD). Pharmacological effects vary, but LSD is believed to act on the serotonergic system. Hallucinogens

---

KEY FACT

Eating large amounts of poppy seed bagels or muffins can result in a urine drug screen that is positive for opioids.

WARDS TIP

Rapid recovery of consciousness following the administration of intravenous (IV) naloxone (opioid antagonist) is consistent with opioid overdose.

KEY FACT

Remember the withdrawal symptoms of opiates: anxiety, insomnia, anorexia, fever, rhinorrhea, piloerection. These are *not* life threatening.

WARDS TIP

Withdrawal from opioids is *not* life threatening, but it does cause severe symptoms.

do not cause physical dependence or withdrawal, though users can rarely develop psychological dependence.

INTOXICATION

- Effects include perceptual changes (illusions, hallucinations, body image distortions, synesthesia), labile affect, dilated pupils, tachycardia, hypertension, hyperthermia, tremors, incoordination, sweating, and palpitations.
- Usually lasts 6–12 hours, but may last for several days.
- May have a "bad trip" that consists of marked anxiety, panic, and psychotic symptoms (paranoia, hallucinations).
- **Treatment**: Monitor for dangerous behavior and reassure patient. Use benzodiazepines first-line (can use antipsychotics) if necessary for agitated psychosis.

WITHDRAWAL

No withdrawal syndrome is produced, but with long-term LSD use, patients may experience "flashbacks" later in life.

Marijuana

- Cannabis ("marijuana," "pot," "weed," "grass") is the most commonly used illicit substance in the world.
- The main active component in cannabis is THC (tetrahydrocannabinol).
- Cannabinoid receptors in the brain inhibit adenylate cyclase.
- Marijuana has shown some efficacy in treating nausea and vomiting in chemotherapy patients, ↑ appetite in AIDS patients, in chronic pain (from cancer), and ↓ intraocular pressure in glaucoma.

INTOXICATION

- Marijuana causes euphoria, anxiety, impaired motor coordination, perceptual disturbances (sensation of slowed time), mild tachycardia, anxiety, **conjunctival injection (red eyes)**, dry mouth, and ↑ appetite ("the munchies").
- Cannabis-induced psychotic disorders with paranoia, hallucinations, and/or delusions may occur. There is no overdose syndrome of marijuana use.
- Cannabis use disorder occurs in approximately 10% of those who use (up to 50% of daily users).
- Chronic use may cause respiratory problems such as asthma and chronic bronchitis, suppression of the immune system, cancer, and possible effects on reproductive hormones.
- **Treatment**: Supportive, psychosocial interventions (e.g., contingency management, groups, etc.).

WITHDRAWAL

- Withdrawal symptoms may include irritability, anxiety, restlessness, aggression, strange dreams, depression, headaches, sweating, chills, insomnia, and ↓ appetite.
- **Treatment**: Supportive and symptomatic.

Inhalants

- Inhalants include a broad range of drugs that are inhaled and absorbed through the lungs.
- Inhalants generally act as CNS depressants.
- User is typically a preadolescent or adolescent; rate of use is similar between boys and girls (but rare in adult females).
- *Examples*: Solvents, glue, paint thinners, fuels, isobutyl nitrates ("huff," "laughing gas," "rush," "bolt").

INTOXICATION

- **Effects**: Perceptual disturbances, paranoia, lethargy, dizziness, nausea/vomiting, headache, nystagmus, tremor, muscle weakness, hyporeflexia, ataxia, slurred speech, euphoria, hypoxia, clouding of consciousness, stupor, or coma.
- Acute intoxication: 15–30 minutes. May be sustained with repeated use.
- **Overdose**: May be fatal secondary to respiratory depression or cardiac arrhythmias.
- Long-term use may cause permanent damage to CNS (e.g., neurocognitive impairment, cerebellar dysfunction, Parkinsonism, seizures), peripheral neuropathy, myopathy, aplastic anemia, malignancy, metabolic acidosis, urinary calculi, glomerulonephritis, myocarditis, myocardial infarction, and hepatotoxicity).
- **Treatment**: Monitor airway, breathing, and circulation; may need oxygen with hypoxic states.
- Identify solvent because some (e.g., leaded gasoline) may require chelation.

WITHDRAWAL

A withdrawal syndrome does not usually occur, but symptoms may include irritability, sleep disturbance, anxiety, depression, nausea, vomiting, and craving.

Caffeine

Caffeine is the most commonly used psychoactive substance in the United States, usually in the form of coffee or tea. It acts as an adenosine antagonist, causing ↑ cyclic adenosine monophosphate (cAMP) and stimulating the release of excitatory neurotransmitters.

OVERDOSE

- >250 mg (2 cups of coffee): Anxiety, insomnia, muscle twitching, rambling speech, flushed face, diuresis, gastrointestinal disturbance, restlessness, excitement, and tachycardia.
- >1 g: May cause tinnitus, severe agitation, visual light flashes, and cardiac arrhythmias.
- >10 g: Death may occur secondary to seizures and respiratory failure.
- **Treatment**: Supportive and symptomatic.

WITHDRAWAL

- Caffeine withdrawal symptoms occur in 50–75% of caffeine users if cessation is abrupt.
- Withdrawal symptoms include **headache**, fatigue, irritability, nausea, vomiting, drowsiness, muscle pain, and depression.
- Usually resolve within 1½ weeks.

Nicotine

- Nicotine is derived from the tobacco plant, and stimulates nicotinic receptors in autonomic ganglia of the sympathetic and parasympathetic nervous systems. It is highly addictive through its effects on the dopaminergic system.
- Smoking → tolerance and physical dependence (i.e., prominent craving and withdrawal).
- Cigarette smoking is the leading cause of preventable morbidity and mortality in the United States, posing many health risks including chronic obstructive pulmonary disease (COPD), cardiovascular diseases, and various cancers.
- Current smoking prevalence is about 21% of US adults.
- Effects: Restlessness, insomnia, anxiety, and ↑ gastrointestinal motility.
- **Withdrawal symptoms**: Intense craving, dysphoria, anxiety, poor concentration, ↑ appetite, weight gain, irritability, restlessness, and insomnia.

WARDS TIP

Cigarette smoking during pregnancy is associated with low birth weight, SIDS, and a variety of postnatal morbidities.

TREATMENT OF NICOTINE DEPENDENCE

FDA-approved pharmacotherapy:

- Varenicline (Chantix): α4β2 nicotinic cholinergic receptor (nAChR) partial agonist that mimics the action of nicotine, reducing the rewarding aspects and preventing withdrawal symptoms.
- Bupropion (Zyban): Antidepressant that is an inhibitor of dopamine and norepinephrine reuptake; helps reduce craving and withdrawal symptoms.
- Nicotine replacement therapy (NRT): Available as transdermal patch, gum, lozenge, nasal spray, and inhaler.
- Behavioral support/counseling should be part of every treatment.
- Relapse after abstinence is common.

Gambling Disorder

DIAGNOSIS AND DSM-5 CRITERIA

Persistent and recurrent problematic gambling behavior, as evidenced by four or more of the following in a 12-month period:

1. Preoccupation with gambling
2. Need to gamble with increasing amount of money to achieve pleasure
3. Repeated and unsuccessful attempts to cut down on or stop gambling
4. Restlessness or irritability when attempting to stop gambling
5. Gambling when feeling distressed (depressed, anxious, etc.)
6. Returning to reclaim losses after gambling ("get even")
7. Lying to hide level of gambling
8. Jeopardizing relationships or job because of gambling
9. Relying on others to financially support gambling

EPIDEMIOLOGY/ETIOLOGY

- Prevalence: 0.4–1.0% of adults in the United States.
- Men represent most of the cases.
- More common in young adults and middle-aged, and lower rates in older adults.
- As similar to substance use disorders, the course is marked by periods of abstinence and relapse.
- ↑ incidence of mood disorders, anxiety disorders, substance use disorders, and personality disorders.
- Etiology may involve genetic, temperamental, environmental, and neuro-chemical factors.
- One-third may achieve recovery without treatment.

TREATMENT

- Participation in Gamblers Anonymous (a 12-step program) is the most common treatment.
- Cognitive behavioral therapy has been shown to be effective, particularly when combined with Gamblers Anonymous.
- Important to treat comorbid mood disorders, anxiety disorders, and substance use disorders as appropriate.

CHAPTER 8

NEUROCOGNITIVE DISORDERS

Definition	98	Diagnosis	102
Delirium	99	Alzheimer's Disease (AD)	104
Epidemiology	99	Vascular Disease (Vascular Cognitive Impairment)	105
Risk Factors	99	Lewy Body Disease (LBD)	106
Etiology	99	Frontotemporal Degeneration (FTD)	107
Clinical Manifestations	99	HIV Infection	108
Diagnosis	100	Huntington's Disease (HD)	108
Treatment	101	Parkinson's Disease (PD)	109
Mild and Major Neurocognitive Disorders	102	Prion Disease	109
		Normal Pressure Hydrocephalus (NPH)	110

Definition

The neurocognitive disorders (NCDs) comprise a group of conditions defined by a decline from a previous level of cognitive functioning. The six cognitive domains that may be affected include **complex attention, executive function, learning and memory, language, perceptual-motor skills**, and **social cognition (interaction)**. By definition, cause(s) for the deficits may be ascertained from findings on history, physical exam, and diagnostic testing. The DSM-5 divides the NCDs into three main categories: delirium, mild NCDs, and major NCDs.

Connie Ang is an 83-year-old woman who was admitted to the general medical hospital after presenting with fever and altered mental status. Her home nurse aide reports that she was in her usual state of health until the day prior to admission, when she was observed to be confused and talking to her mother, who died almost 20 years ago. Reportedly, her mental status improved to near baseline within a few hours. However, the nurse aide later called the ambulance because Mrs. Ang was observed dialing 911, stating that people were in her house trying to kill her. On examination, Mrs. Ang is somnolent, has difficulty concentrating, and requires questions to be repeated frequently. She is restless, paranoid, and disoriented to place and time. She is observed to be addressing the chair in the room as her mother and appears to be gesturing and calling her dog to come and sit next to her.

Mrs. Ang's daughter states that she has had progressive memory deficits. Family members report that she initially confused her grandchildren's names and had difficulty remembering recent conversations with them. They report that her symptoms have worsened over the past several years. As an example, they describe an episode during which she forgot to turn off the stove, almost burning her house down. She requires assistance managing her finances, driving, and preparing meals, but is independent in basic self-care activities. Due to this, Mrs. Ang has had a 24-hour home health aide for the past 2 years.

What is her most likely diagnosis?

Mrs. Ang's most likely diagnosis is delirium. She presents with a sudden change in cognition as manifested by inattention, confusion, disorientation, and hallucinations. She has had an acute change from her baseline behavior, and her symptoms have waxed and waned throughout the day, representing the typical fluctuation of symptoms found in delirium. Mrs. Ang presented with a fever, likely secondary to an infection, which is the most likely cause of her symptoms. If this were confirmed, her diagnosis would then be identified as delirium due to the specific infectious etiology.

Collateral information obtained from family members points to a prior diagnosis of major neurocognitive disorder (dementia). Mrs. Ang has a history of memory impairment that began gradually and has progressively worsened. There is also history of impairment in executive functioning, and she can no longer care for herself. The existence of a major neurocognitive disorder is a risk factor for the development of a superimposed delirium.

Delirium

> A 70-year-old woman presents to the emergency department with increasing confusion over the past 24 hours. Her son reports that she has been sleeping much more than usual and that she is irritable when awoken. On exam, she is lethargic, inattentive, and disoriented to time. Exam reveals suprapubic discomfort to palpation. *What is the likely etiology of this patient's delirium?* UTI.

- Delirium is a **medical emergency**. It may be the only early manifestation of serious illness.
- Reversible, but can potentially advance to coma, seizures, or death.
- Associated with **high mortality**. Up to 40% of individuals die within 1 year of diagnosis.

EPIDEMIOLOGY

- As many as 50% of medically admitted patients develop delirium.
- Delirium often goes unrecognized.

RISK FACTORS

- Polypharmacy, including the use of psychotropic medications (especially benzodiazepines and anticholinergic drugs).
- Advanced age.
- Preexisting cognitive impairment or depression.
- Prior history of delirium.
- Alcohol use.
- Severe or terminal illness.
- Multiple medical comorbidities.
- Impaired mobility.
- Hearing or vision impairment.
- Malnutrition.
- Male gender.
- Pain.

ETIOLOGY

- Almost any medical condition can cause delirium (see examples in Table 8-1).
- The DSM-5 recognizes five broad categories:
    - Substance intoxication delirium
    - Substance withdrawal delirium
    - Medication-induced delirium
    - Delirium due to another medical condition
    - Delirium due to multiple etiologies

CLINICAL MANIFESTATIONS

- Primarily a disorder of **attention** and **awareness** (i.e., **orientation**).
- Cognitive deficits **develop acutely** over hours to days.
- Symptoms **fluctuate** throughout the course of a day, typically worsening at night.

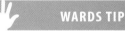

WARDS TIP

The ICU triad includes delirium, pain, and agitation. All three of these interdependent conditions must be addressed.

WARDS TIP

Think of delirium as acute brain failure—a *medical emergency* like other acute organ failures.

WARDS TIP

Terms commonly used for delirium include *toxic or metabolic encephalopathy, acute organic brain syndrome, acute confusional state, acute toxic psychosis,* and *ICU psychosis.*

WARDS TIP

Delirium is common in intensive care and postoperative settings.

WARDS TIP

Common causes of medication-induced delirium:
- Tricyclic antidepressants
- Anticholinergics
- Benzodiazepines
- Nonbenzodiazepine hypnotics ("Z-drugs")
- Corticosteroids
- H2 blockers
- Meperidine

TABLE 8-1. Clinical Scenarios of Delirium on Exam

SCENARIO	LIKELY DIAGNOSIS	DIAGNOSTIC TESTING
Delirium + hemiparesis or other focal neurological signs and symptoms	CVA or mass lesion	Head CT/Brain MRI
Delirium + elevated blood pressure + papilledema	Hypertensive encephalopathy	Head CT/Brain MRI
Delirium + dilated pupils + tachycardia	Drug intoxication	Urine toxicology screen
Delirium + fever + nuchal rigidity + photophobia	Meningitis	Lumbar puncture
Delirium + tachycardia + tremor + thyromegaly	Thyrotoxicosis	Free T_4, T_3, TSH

- Other features include deficits in **recent memory**, language abnormalities, or perceptual disturbances (usually **visual**, such as illusions or hallucinations).
- Circadian rhythm disruption and emotional symptoms are common.
- There are three types of delirium based on psychomotor activity.
  - Mixed type
    - Psychomotor activity may remain stable at baseline or fluctuate rapidly between hyperactivity and hypoactivity.
    - **Most common** type.
  - Hypoactive ("quiet") type
    - Decreased psychomotor activity, ranging from drowsiness to lethargy to stupor.
    - **More likely to go undetected.**
    - More common in the elderly.
  - Hyperactive type ("ICU psychosis")
    - Manifests with agitation, mood lability, and uncooperativeness.
    - Less common, but more easily identified due to its disruptiveness.
    - More common in **drug withdrawal or toxicity**.
- Complete recovery occurs in most hospitalized patients within about 1 week; however, some cognitive deficits can persist for months or even remain indefinitely.

DIAGNOSIS

- Table 8-2 summarizes the DSM-5 diagnostic criteria.
- A useful clinical tool for evaluation of a patient with suspected delirium is the **Confusion Assessment Method (CAM)**.
  - This method takes only 5 minutes to perform and has a high sensitivity and specificity.
  - Delirium is diagnosed in a patient with **inattention** of **acute onset** and/or **fluctuating course** along with either **disorganized thinking** or **altered consciousness**.
    - Inattention manifests as distractibility or difficulty maintaining focus during the evaluation.

TABLE 8-2. DSM-5 Criteria for Delirium

- Disturbance in **attention** and **awareness**.

- Disturbance in **an additional cognitive domain**.

- Develops **acutely** over hours to days, represents a **change** from baseline, and tends to **fluctuate**.

- **Not** better accounted for by **another neurocognitive disorder**.

- **Not** occurring during a **coma**.

- Evidence from history, physical, or labs that the disturbance is a **direct consequence** of **another medical condition**, **substance intoxication/withdrawal**, exposure to **toxin**, or due to multiple etiologies.

- Disorganized thinking is demonstrated via derailment or loose associations.
- Level of consciousness ranges from vigilant (hyperalert) to alert (normal) to lethargic (drowsy, but easily aroused) to stuporous (difficult to arouse) to comatose (unarousable to verbal stimulation).
- Once delirium has been diagnosed, the cause(s) should be sought.
  - Finger-stick blood glucose, pulse-oximetry, arterial blood gases, and electrocardiography can quickly provide useful data at bedside.
  - Labs typically obtained in a delirium workup include a basic metabolic panel, complete blood count with differential, urinalysis, and urine culture.
  - Urine drug screen, a blood alcohol level, therapeutic drug levels (e.g., antiepileptics, digoxin, lithium), a hepatic panel, thyroid hormone levels, or a chest x-ray may also be warranted depending on the clinical presentation.
  - Head imaging (head CT or MRI brain), EEG, and lumbar puncture should be performed if focal neurological deficits are present or a cause of delirium cannot be identified with the initial workup.

TREATMENT

- **Treat the underlying cause(s).**
- Address potential exacerbating factors, such as mobility limitations, sensory deficits, sleep cycle disruption, constipation, urinary retention, dehydration and electrolyte abnormalities, uncontrolled pain, and use of unnecessary medications.
- Encourage a family member to stay at bedside to provide company and redirection as needed.
- Maintain adequate supervision, utilizing a one-to-one sitter if necessary.
- Reorient the patient on a regular basis by drawing attention to time, place, and situation and by keeping whiteboards, calendars, and clocks in plain sight.
- D2 antagonists (i.e., antipsychotics) are indicated for treatment of agitation that places the patient or others at risk.
- **Haloperidol** is the preferred agent and can be administered orally, intramuscularly, or intravenously.
- D2 antagonists exacerbate extrapyramidal symptoms, so use with caution in patients with Parkinsonism.

WARDS TIP

Consider head CT for a patient with delirium under the following circumstances:
- No underlying cause is evident on initial evaluation.
- The delirium occurs in the context of head trauma.
- New focal neurologic deficits are detected on exam.
- The patient in unable or unwilling to cooperate with neurologic examination.
- No improvement occurs despite treatment of already identified causes.

- Benzodiazepines can cause, worsen, or prolong delirium, so do not use unless treating delirium due to alcohol or benzodiazepine withdrawal.
- Avoid the use of restraints, which may worsen agitation and cause injury.
- If restraints are necessary, use the least restrictive means appropriate for the situation, and remove them as soon as the patient meets criteria for release.

WARDS TIP

Avoid using benzodiazepines to treat delirium that is not due to alcohol or benzodiazepine withdrawal. These medications often worsen delirium by causing paradoxical disinhibition or oversedation.

Mild and Major Neurocognitive Disorders

- The non-delirium NCDs are characterized by a more chronic cognitive decline that impacts functioning in daily activities (Table 8-3).
- Individuals with **mild NCDs** (aka mild cognitive impairment) experience difficulty with some of the more complex activities of daily living, but are able to maintain their independence.
- Patients with **major NCDs** require assistance with independent activities of daily living (IADLs), such as paying bills, managing medications, or shopping for groceries. Over time, the basic activities of daily living (e.g., feeding, toileting, bathing) are affected, eventually leading to total dependence.
- The mild and major NCDs are also subcategorized by etiology (Table 8-4).
  - The **dementias** comprise a large group of progressive and irreversible major NCDs that primarily affect the elderly.
  - Several other major NCDs present similarly to the dementias, but their progression may be halted or even reversed with treatment (e.g., vitamin B_{12} deficiency, thyroid dysfunction, normal pressure hydrocephalus).

DIAGNOSIS

- The **Mini Mental State Exam (MMSE)** is a screening test used due to its speed and ease of administration (see Table 8-5).

TABLE 8-3.   DSM-5 Criteria for Mild and Major NCDs

CRITERION	MILD NCDs	MAJOR NCDs
Functional decline in at least 1 cognitive domain relative to baseline as evidenced by		
Concern (expressed by the patient or someone who knows them)	Mild decline	Significant decline
Objective findings on cognitive testing (preferably standardized neuropsychological testing)	Modest impairment	Substantial impairment
Effect on functioning in daily life.	Ability to perform IADLs preserved	Impaired performance of IADLs/ADLs
Deficits do not occur exclusively in the context of a delirium.		
Deficits are not better explained by another mental disorder.		

Note: IADLs, independent activities of daily living; ADLs, basic activities of daily living.

TABLE 8-4. **Clinical Scenarios of Mild or Major Neurocognitive Disorder on Exam**

Scenario	Likely Diagnosis	Diagnostic Testing
Cognitive impairment with stepwise ↑ in severity + focal neurological signs	Vascular disease	Head CT/Brain MRI
Cognitive impairment + cogwheel rigidity + resting tremor	Lewy body disease Parkinson's disease	Clinical
Cognitive impairment + gait apraxia + urinary incontinence + dilated cerebral ventricles	Normal pressure hydrocephalus	Head CT/Brain MRI
Cognitive impairment + fatigue + cold intolerance + coarse hair + constipation	Hypothyroidism	TSH, free T_4
Cognitive impairment + paresthesias + diminished position and vibration sensation + megaloblasts on CBC	Vitamin B_{12} deficiency	Serum B_{12}
Cognitive impairment + tremor + Kayser–Fleischer rings + abnormal LFTs	Wilson's disease	Ceruloplasmin
Cognitive impairment + diminished position and vibration sensation + **A**rgyll **R**obertson **P**upils (**A**ccommodation **R**esponse **P**resent, response to light absent)	Neurosyphilis	CSF FTA-ABS and VDRL

Note: CBC, complete blood count; CSF, cerebrospinal fluid; CT, computed tomography; FTA-ABS, fluorescent treponemal antibody absorption test; LFT, liver function test; MRI, magnetic resonance imaging; T_4, thyroxine; TSH, thyroid-stimulating hormone; VDRL, Venereal Disease Research Laboratory.

- Assesses orientation, attention/concentration, language, constructional ability, and immediate and delayed recall.
- Sensitive for major NCDs (e.g., dementias), particularly moderate-to-severe forms.
  - Perfect score: 30
  - Dysfunction: <25
- Not as sensitive for mild NCDs and early major NCDs.
- Lacks specificity.
- Norm tables are available to adjust for age and education.
- Another commonly used screening tool is the **Mini-Cog**.
  - Consists of 3-item recall and clock-drawing tasks.
  - Positive screening for cognitive impairment:
    - No items recalled after 3 minutes.
    - Only one to two items recalled with abnormal clock drawing.
  - Negative screening:
    - All three items repeated correctly after 3 minutes.
    - One to two items recalled with normal clock drawing.
- Other commonly used screening tools include:
  - Blessed Orientation-Memory-Concentration (BOMC)
  - Montreal Cognitive Assessment (MoCA)
  - Frontal Assessment Battery (FAB)
- An abnormal screening test indicates the need for further testing, preferably formal neuropsychological testing.

KEY FACT

Thyroid dysfunction can cause reversible cognitive impairment. Hypothyroidism is typically accompanied by fatigue and cold intolerance. Hyperthyroidism in the elderly may manifest as an "apathetic thyrotoxicosis," characterized by depression and lethargy. Thyroid function tests are typically included in the initial evaluation of any psychiatric illness.

TABLE 8-5.   **Performing the Mini-Mental State Exam**

1. Orientation (Awareness)	
What is the date (day of week, day of month, month, season, and year)?	5 points
Where are we (state, county, city, hospital, and floor)?	5 points
2. Registration	
Name three objects and repeat them.	3 points
3. Attention	
Serial 7s (subtract 7 from 100 and continue subtracting 7 from each answer) or spell "world" backward.	5 points
4. Recall (Recent Memory)	
Name the three objects above 5 minutes later.	3 points
5. Language	
Naming: Name a pen and a clock.	2 points
Repetition: Say, "No ifs, ands, or buts."	1 points
Verbal comprehension (three-step command): Take a pencil in your right hand, put in your left hand, then put it on the floor.	3 points
Written comprehension: Read the statement written on a piece of paper, and do what it says: "Close your eyes."	1 point
Writing: Write a sentence.	1 point
Visuospatial skills: Draw two intersecting pentagons.	1 point
TOTAL	**30 points**

ALZHEIMER'S DISEASE (AD)

- Alzheimer's disease is the **most common** underlying etiology of major NCDs (dementias).

Clinical Manifestations

- **Gradual progressive decline** in cognitive functions.
- The primary cognitive domains affected are **memory**, **learning**, and **language**.
- Personality changes, mood swings, and paranoia are very common.
- Motor and sensory symptoms are absent until late in the course of the illness.
- On average, death occurs 10 years after diagnosis.

Diagnosis

- Definitive diagnosis can only be established postmortem.
- A diagnosis of **possible** NCD due to AD is made based on the presence of characteristic clinical findings:
    - Insidious onset.
    - Gradual progression.
    - Impairment in one (mild NCD) or more (major NCD) cognitive domains.
- NCD due to AD is **probable** if there is evidence of causation by one of several single-gene variants.

Etiology

- Accumulation of extraneuronal *beta*-amyloid plaques and intraneuronal *tau* protein tangles is associated with progressive brain atrophy.
- Approximately 1% of AD results from an autosomal dominant single-gene mutation (amyloid precursor protein, presenilin 1, or presenilin 2), which results in an early onset of symptoms.
- Having the *epsilon*-4 variant of the *apolipoprotein* gene is also a risk factor for developing early-onset AD.

Epidemiology

- AD pathology is estimated to play a role in 60–90% of major NCDs.
- Approximately 50% of patients with AD pathology actually have an NCD due to multiple etiologies.
- $^2/_3$ of patients diagnosed with AD are women.
- Diagnosed after the age of 65 in the vast majority of individuals.

Treatment

- No cure or truly effective treatment.
- **Cholinesterase inhibitors**, such as donepezil, rivastigmine, and galantamine, may slow clinical deterioration by 6–12 months in up to 50% of patients with mild-to-moderate AD.
- The **NMDA receptor antagonist**, memantine, may provide a modest benefit to patients with moderate-to-severe disease.
- Antipsychotic medications are often used to treat agitation and aggression.
    - Because they are associated with **increased mortality** in patients with dementia, low doses should be prescribed for short periods of time.
    - Ideally, informed consent should be obtained from patients and/or their designated decision makers.
    - **Monitor closely** for side effects.
- Supportive care via behavioral, social, and environmental interventions.
- A **multidisciplinary approach** is necessary.
- Any treatment plan must include **caregiver support**.

VASCULAR DISEASE (VASCULAR COGNITIVE IMPAIRMENT)

A 68-year-old woman is brought to the clinic by her husband. He reports that she has recently seemed confused and has been crying at the slightest provocation. The patient is able to complete her daily activities at home, but reports some increased difficulty with planning and decision-making. Her medical history is significant for hypertension and transient ischemic attacks (TIAs). A physical exam reveals a carotid bruit.

What is the likely diagnosis? Mild vascular NCD.

KEY FACT

Senile plaques and neurofibrillary tangles are found in Alzheimer's disease, but also in Down syndrome and even normal aging.

KEY FACT

Postmortem pathological examination of the brain is the only way to definitively diagnose Alzheimer's disease.

KEY FACT

Adults with Down syndrome are at ↑ risk of developing Alzheimer's disease in midlife.

WARDS TIP

Antipsychotics carry a black box warning regarding increased risk of death in patients with dementia.

A lesion to the frontal lobe can manifest with a spectrum of symptoms including personality changes, disinhibition, inappropriate behavior, aggression, apathy, amotivation, and paranoia.

Classically, patients with vascular NCDs have a stepwise loss of function corresponding with the occurrence of micro-infarcts (multi-infarct dementia).

- Second most common single cause of major NCD after AD, accounting for approximately 20% of major NCDs.
- Evidence of vascular disease is found in $\frac{1}{2}$ of all major NCDs, most commonly comorbid with AD pathology (NCD due to multiple etiologies).
- Cognitive decline occurs as a result of at least one of the following mechanisms:
  - Large vessel strokes, usually cortical.
  - Small vessel strokes (lacunar infarcts) to subcortical structures.
  - Microvascular disease affecting the periventricular white matter.
- Effects vary based on the size, location, and number of infarcts.

Risk Factors

- Hypertension
- Diabetes
- Smoking
- Obesity
- Hyperlipidemia
- Atrial fibrillation
- Old age

Clinical Manifestations

- Presentation and progression of cognitive impairment are variable.
  - Classically demonstrates a stepwise deterioration.
  - May present with acute onset followed by partial improvement.
  - May have an insidious onset with gradual decline similar to AD.
- **Complex attention** and **executive functions** are the cognitive domains typically affected in small vessel disease.
- Confirmation of the diagnosis requires neuroimaging with findings that correlate to the clinical picture.

Treatment

- No cure or truly effective treatment.
- Manage risk factors with a goal of preventing future strokes.
- Symptomatic treatment is similar to AD.

LEWY BODY DISEASE (LBD)

- As reflected in its name, the major pathologic features of LBD are Lewy bodies (pathologic aggregations of *alpha*-synuclein) and Lewy neurites in the brain, primarily in the basal ganglia.

Clinical Manifestations

- Progressive cognitive decline.
- Core features:
  - **Waxing and waning** of cognition, especially in the areas of **attention** and **alertness**.
  - **Visual hallucinations**—usually vivid, colorful, well-formed images of animals or small people.
  - Development of **extrapyramidal signs** (Parkinsonism) at least 1 year after cognitive decline becomes evident.
- Suggestive features:
  - **Rapid eye movement (REM) sleep behavior disorder**—violent movements during sleep in response to dreams, often of fighting.
  - Pronounced **antipsychotic sensitivity**.
- Commonly coexists with AD and/or cerebrovascular disease as NCD due to multiple etiologies.

Diagnosis

- Definitive diagnosis can only be made with autopsy.
- **Possible** NCD with Lewy bodies: Only 1 core feature or ≥1 suggestive feature.
- **Probable** NCD with Lewy bodies: ≥2 core features OR 1 core feature and ≥1 suggestive feature.

Treatment

- **Cholinesterase inhibitors** for cognitive and behavioral symptoms.
- **Quetiapine** or **clozapine** for psychotic symptoms.
    - Use the lowest effective dose for the shortest period of time possible.
    - Monitor closely for adverse effects, such as extrapyramidal signs, sedation, increased confusion, autonomic dysfunction, and signs of **Neuroleptic Malignant Syndrome (NMS)**.
- Levodopa-carbidopa for Parkinsonism.
    - Not as effective as in idiopathic Parkinson's disease.
    - May exacerbate psychosis or REM sleep behavior disorder.
- Melatonin and/or clonazepam for REM sleep behavior disorder.

FRONTOTEMPORAL DEGENERATION (FTD)

- FTD includes a diverse group of clinical and pathological disorders that typically present between the ages of 45 and 65.
- Approximately 40% are familial, and 10% are autosomal dominant.

Clinical Manifestations

- Cognitive deficits in **attention, abstraction, planning,** and **problem solving**.
- **Behavioral variant:**
    - **Disinhibited** verbal, physical, or sexual behavior.
    - Overeating or oral exploration of inanimate objects.
    - Lack of emotional warmth, empathy, or sympathy.
    - Apathy or inertia.
    - Perseveration, repetitive speech, rituals, or obsessions.
    - Decline in **social cognition** and/or **executive abilities**.
- **Language variant** (primary progressive aphasia):
    - Difficulties with **speech** and **comprehension**.
- Relative sparing of learning/memory and perceptual-motor function.
- Many individuals have features of both the behavioral and language variants.
- Increased sensitivity to adverse effects of antipsychotics.

Pathology

- Marked atrophy of the frontal and temporal lobes.

Diagnosis

- Definitive diagnosis cannot be made until autopsy.
- FTD is **probable** if frontotemporal atrophy is evident on structural imaging or hypoactivity is visualized on functional imaging in context of the characteristic clinical signs.

Treatment

- Symptom-focused.
- Serotonergic medications (e.g., SSRIs, trazodone) may help reduce disinhibition, anxiety, impulsivity, repetitive behaviors, and eating disorders.

HIV INFECTION

- HIV is the most common infectious agent known to cause cognitive impairment.
- 25% of persons infected with HIV meet mild NCD criteria and <5% meet major NCD criteria.

Risk Factors

- History of severe immunosuppression.
- High viral loads in the CSF.
- Advanced HIV infection.

Clinical Manifestations

- Variable presentation depending on the part(s) of the brain affected.
- Decline may be observed in executive functioning, attention, working memory, and psychomotor activity.
- Psychiatric and neuromotor symptoms may also be present.

Diagnosis

- Mild or major NCD attributable to confirmed HIV infection.

Treatment

- Highly active antiretroviral therapy (HAART) improves cognition in some patients.
- Psychostimulants target fatigue, apathy, and psychomotor retardation.

HUNTINGTON'S DISEASE (HD)

- A genetic disorder resulting from trinucleotide (CAG) repeats in the gene encoding the huntingtin (HTT) protein on chromosome 4.
- Autosomal dominant mode of inheritance.

Clinical Manifestations

- Characterized by a triad of **motor**, **cognitive**, and **psychiatric** symptoms.
- Average age at diagnosis is 40 years.
- Cognitive decline and behavioral changes can precede onset of motor signs by up to 15 years.
- **Executive function** is the primary cognitive domain affected.
- Psychiatric manifestations include depression, apathy, irritability, obsessions, and impulsivity.
- Patients are often aware of deteriorating mentation.
- ↑ rate of suicide.
- Movement disorders include **chorea** (jerky, dance-like movements) and **bradykinesia**.

Diagnosis

- Extrapyramidal movement disorder in an individual with either a **family history** of HD or **genetic testing** that confirms an increased number of CAG repeats in the HTT gene.
- Mild or major NCD due to HD may be diagnosed prior to onset of motor signs if an individual is determined to be at risk based on family history or genetic testing.

Treatment

- Symptom-directed therapy, with **tetrabenazine** or **atypical (second-generation) antipsychotics**.

PARKINSON'S DISEASE (PD)

- An idiopathic, progressive neurodegenerative disease characterized by depletion of dopamine in the basal ganglia.
- Up to 75% of patients with PD meet the criteria for major NCD, typically late in the course of the disease.

Clinical Manifestations

- Motor signs include rigidity, resting tremor, bradykinesia, and postural instability.
- Cognitive manifestations consist of executive dysfunction and visuospatial impairments.
- Depression, anxiety, personality changes, and apathy are common.
- Psychotic symptoms, including visual hallucinations and paranoid delusions, may result from the disease itself or as adverse effects of medications used to treat the motor symptoms.

Diagnosis

- Diagnosis of PD requires the presence of **bradykinesia** and either **tremor** or **rigidity**.
- Asymmetry of motor symptoms and favorable response to dopaminergic therapy support the diagnosis.
- Mild or major NCD is attributed to PD if **cognitive decline appears after the onset of motor symptoms** and no other underlying etiology is identified.

Treatment

- Motor symptoms are most commonly treated with **carbidopa-levodopa** and/or **dopamine agonists**.
- Cholinesterase inhibitors are used to target cognitive symptoms and may also ameliorate some of the neuropsychiatric symptoms (hallucinations).
- Psychotic symptoms may respond to a reduction in the dose of dopamine agonists.
- **Quetiapine** and **clozapine** are the preferred medications for treatment of psychotic symptoms that are not responsive to dose reduction. Other antipsychotics should be avoided, as they tend to exacerbate the motor symptoms of PD.

KEY FACT

Symptoms of Parkinson's disease can be exacerbated by antipsychotic medications.

PRION DISEASE

- A form of subacute spongiform encephalopathy caused by *pro*teinaceous *in*fectious particles (prions).
- Most cases occur sporadically.
- The most common type is **Creutzfeldt–Jakob disease**.
- Up to 15% are familial (autosomal dominant).
- <1% are iatrogenic.

Clinical Manifestations

- Insidious onset with **rapidly progressive** cognitive decline.
- Difficulties with **concentration**, **memory**, and **judgment** occur early.

- More than 90% of patients experience **myoclonus** (often provoked by startle) at some point in the illness.
- Depression, apathy, and hypersomnia are also common.
- Basal ganglia and cerebellar dysfunction, manifesting as **ataxia, nystagmus,** and **hypokinesia,** are present in a majority of individuals.

Diagnosis

- Definitive diagnosis requires analysis of brain tissue obtained via biopsy or autopsy.
- A diagnosis of probable CJD requires:
  - **Rapid progression** of cognitive decline.
  - At least two of the following typical clinical features.
    - **Myoclonus.**
    - Visual or cerebellar signs.
    - Pyramidal or extrapyramidal signs.
    - Akinetic mutism.
  - Supportive findings from at least one diagnostic modality.
    - Periodic sharp wave complexes on EEG.
    - CSF positive for 14-3-3 proteins.
    - Lesions in the putamen or caudate nucleus on MRI.

Treatment

- No effective treatment exists.
- Most individuals die within 1 year of diagnosis.

NORMAL PRESSURE HYDROCEPHALUS (NPH)

- NPH is a potentially reversible cause of cognitive dysfunction.
- Enlarged ventricles (on imaging) with a localized elevation of cerebrospinal fluid (CSF) pressure but normal opening pressures on lumbar puncture.
- The etiology is either idiopathic or secondary to obstruction of CSF reabsorption sites due to infection (meningitis) or hemorrhage (subarachnoid or intraventricular).

Clinical Manifestations

- Classically presents with a clinical triad:
  - **Gait disturbance** ("Wobbly")
    - Most likely to be the first manifestation.
    - Slow with short steps.
    - Broad-based with outwardly rotated feet.
    - Feet appear to be stuck to the floor.
    - Postural instability leads to recurrent falls.
    - Most responsive to treatment.
  - **Urinary incontinence** ("Wet")
    - May begin as urinary urgency.
    - Gait disturbance may interfere with reaching the toilet before loss of urine.
    - In later stages, apathy may contribute.
  - **Cognitive impairment** ("Wacky")
    - Insidious onset.
    - Executive dysfunction.
    - Psychomotor retardation.
    - Decreased attention.
    - Apathy.

- Neuroimaging shows enlargement of ventricles out of proportion to cortical atrophy.
- Clinical improvement with CSF removal via lumbar puncture is supportive of the diagnosis.

Treatment

- Placement of a shunt (usually ventriculoperitoneal) may improve symptoms.
- Of the clinical triad, the cognitive impairment is least likely to improve.

CHAPTER 9

GERIATRIC PSYCHIATRY

Normal Aging	114
Major Depression	114
Pseudodementia	114
TREATMENT	114
Bereavement	117
Substance Use	117
Psychiatric Manifestations of Major Neurocognitive Disorders (Dementia)	118
TREATMENT	118
Sleep Disturbance	119
Other Issues	120
RESTRAINTS	120
MEDICATIONS	120
ELDER ABUSE	120
NURSING HOMES	120

The geriatric population of the United States is projected to more than double by the year 2050, boosted in a large part by the aging Baby Boomer generation. Nearly 20% of people over the age of 60 have a psychiatric disorder. The suicide rate of elderly (aged 85 and older) white men is five times the national average.

Common diagnoses in elderly patients include mood disorders, anxiety disorders, and neurocognitive disorders, though many mental disorders in this population remain underreported.

Normal Aging

Factors associated with normal aging include:

- ↓ brain weight/enlarged ventricles and sulci
- ↓ muscle mass/↑ fat
- Impaired vision and hearing
- Minor forgetfulness (sometimes called age-associated memory impairment or benign senescent forgetfulness)

Major Depression

WARDS TIP

Work up an elderly patient for major depression when he or she presents with memory loss or nonspecific physical complaints.

Major depression is a common mental disorder in the geriatric population, with depressive symptoms present in 5–15% of the elderly. Depression is associated with poor physical health:

- Post-myocardial infarction (MI) patients who develop depression have a 4× ↑ rate of death.
- Stroke patients who develop depression have >3× ↑ rate of death during the 10 years following their stroke.
- New admits to nursing homes suffering from depression have an ↑ 1-year mortality rate.

Pseudodementia

WARDS TIP

Patients with a major neurocognitive disorder are more likely to confabulate when they do not know an answer, whereas depressed patients may just say that they don't know. When pressed for an answer, depressed patients will often show the capacity to answer correctly.

Symptoms of major depression in the elderly often include problems with memory and cognitive functioning. Because this clinical picture may be mistaken for a major neurocognitive disorder (dementia), it is termed *pseudodementia*.

Pseudodementia is the presence of apparent cognitive deficits in patients with major depression. Patients may appear demented. However, their symptoms are only secondary to their underlying depression, and it can be difficult to differentiate the two (see Table 9-1).

TREATMENT

- Supportive psychotherapy.
- Community resources: Senior centers, senior services, support groups, etc.
- Low-dose antidepressant medication (selective serotonin reuptake inhibitors [SSRIs] have the fewest side effects and are generally preferable to tricyclic antidepressants [TCAs] or monoamine oxidase [MAO] inhibitors).

TABLE 9-1. **Dementia Versus Pseudodementia (Depression)**

DEMENTIA	PSEUDODEMENTIA (DEPRESSION)
Onset is insidious.	Onset is more acute.
Sundowning is common (↑ confusion at night).	Sundowning is uncommon.
Will guess at answers (confabulate).	Often answers "I don't know."
Patient is unaware of problems.	Patient is aware of problems.
Cognitive deficits do not improve with antidepressant treatment.	Cognitive deficits improve with antidepressants.

- If using TCAs in elderly patients, nortriptyline is favored because it has the fewest anticholinergic side effects.
- Mirtazapine can ↑ appetite and is also sedating; it is often dosed at bedtime for depressed patients who also suffer from ↓ appetite and sleep disturbances.
- Methylphenidate can be used at low doses as an adjunct to antidepressants for patients with severe depression and/or psychomotor retardation; however, it may cause insomnia if given in the afternoon or evening. Also be aware of arrhythmia risks in cardiac patients.
- Electroconvulsive therapy (ECT) may be used in place of antidepressants (safe and effective in the elderly).

WARDS TIP

The elderly are very sensitive to side effects of medications, particularly anticholinergic effects of antidepressants.

Mrs. Brennan is a 72-year-old Caucasian woman who considers herself to be in good health. She goes out to lunch with friends three times a week and looks forward to her Saturday bridge games at the local senior center. Unfortunately, her husband has suffered from years of ill health, including five myocardial infarctions and a serious stroke last year that left him barely able to walk. You are a geriatric psychiatrist who has been treating Mrs. Brennan's husband for depression that began after his last stroke. Mrs. Brennan always comes along to appointments so that she can stay informed about her husband's medical care.

You become concerned when your patient uncharacteristically misses an appointment and does not return your phone message. Finally, a month later, you are surprised to see Mrs. Brennan walk into your office alone. She enters the room slowly, and you notice that she has lost some weight since you last saw her.

She sits down but does not make eye contact. Finally, she begins to talk in a soft, monotone voice, explaining that her husband had another bad stroke last month and was moved to a hospice facility, where he passed away 2 weeks ago. She begins to cry, and you hand her some tissues. The two of you talk some more about her husband's death and how she is coping with it. She reports that her daughter visits her frequently and has invited her to spend the weekends with her.

Although Mrs. Brennan reports that she feels "down," she reports that she is making an effort to go on with her life because that is what her husband would have wanted. She says that she went out to lunch with her friends this week and adds that they are very supportive. Mrs. Brennan also reports that it is difficult for her to realize that her husband is no longer there and says that she has heard his voice calling her a couple of times this week. As she leaves your office, you tell her she is welcome to come back whenever she wants.

Is Mrs. Brennan having a normal grief reaction?

Yes, Mrs. Brennan is going through a normal grieving process, also known as bereavement. Although she displays some symptoms suggestive of major depression (psychomotor retardation, depressed mood), and reports the presence of auditory hallucinations (her husband's voice), these symptoms are commonly encountered in bereavement and are considered a normal reaction to her sudden loss.

Three months later, you receive a phone call from Mrs. Brennan's daughter, who expresses concern about her mother. She tells you that her mother has to be urged to shower, wear clean clothes, and eat regularly. Mrs. Brennan has stopped participating in her bridge group and has not been out with her friends in many weeks. The daughter also worries about Mrs. Brennan's increasing forgetfulness and memory problems. She asks if she can bring her in for an appointment with you. You agree immediately and schedule Mrs. Brennan the next day.

Mrs. Brennan enters your office with her daughter by her side. She is dressed in a wrinkled pantsuit and is wearing scuffed shoes. Her hair is clean but lies limply against her head. She appears much thinner than the last time you saw her. Her eyes are downcast, and she appears sad. You try to engage her in conversation, but her answers to your questions are soft and short. When you do an assessment of her memory, you note that she answers basic questions with "I don't know" and scores poorly on the mini-mental state exam questions.

What is Mrs. Brennan's most likely diagnosis now?

Mrs. Brennan is most likely suffering from a major depressive episode. Her symptoms now fulfill criteria for major depressive disorder and have been present for over 2 weeks. Since her memory problems began after she began experiencing depressive symptoms, these are most likely secondary to depression. When this occurs, it is often referred to as "pseudodementia." If this is the case, as her depression is treated, her memory deficits will improve.

What are possible treatment options for Mrs. Brennan?

Supportive psychotherapy and a medication trial of a low-dose SSRI would be excellent first-line treatments. In addition, you suggest to Mrs. Brennan and her daughter to consider visiting her local senior center to learn what kinds of services she might benefit from.

Bereavement

In 1969, Elisabeth Kübler-Ross, MD, published a book called *On Death and Dying*, in which she proposed a model of bereavement, the Five Stages of Grief.

- **Denial:** *"This isn't happening to me. I don't feel sick."*
- **Anger:** *"It's my ex-husband's fault for smoking around me all those years!"*
- **Bargaining:** *"Maybe if I exercise and improve my diet, I'll get better."*
- **Depression:** *"There's no hope for a cure. I will die of this cancer."*
- **Acceptance:** *"I may have cancer, but I've always been a fighter—why stop now?"*

There is some controversy surrounding this model (e.g., people may not experience all of the stages or they may go through them in a different order) as grief is a very individualized experience; there is no "correct" way to mourn a loss. However, it is important to be able to distinguish normal grief reactions from unhealthy, pathological ones.

- **Normal grief** may involve many intense feelings, including guilt and sadness, sleep disturbances, appetite changes, and illusions (not always pathological in some cultures). These feelings generally abate within 6 months of the loss, and the patient's ability to function appropriately in their life is preserved.
- **Bereavement-associated depression** is major depression that began with a concrete death or loss in the patient's life. It is often difficult to distinguish between depression and grief, since many symptoms are similar.
  - Look for generalized feelings of hopelessness, helplessness, severe guilt and worthlessness, neurovegetative symptoms (e.g., insomnia, appetite/weight changes, low energy), and suicidal ideation, in addition to grief symptoms.
  - Treatment for depression is recommended in patients who have 2 straight weeks of depressive symptoms.

Substance Use

- 40% of the 65+-year-old population drinks alcohol, and up to 16% are heavy drinkers who may experience adverse health events from the amount of alcohol they use or from its interaction with medications and impact on chronic disease processes.
- Age-related effects of alcohol:
  - ↓ alcohol dehydrogenase can → higher blood alcohol levels (BALs) with fewer drinks as compared to younger adults
  - ↓ amount of water in the body with age, resulting in a higher percentage of alcohol in their blood compared to younger people after drinking the same amount of alcohol
  - ↑ central nervous system sensitivity to alcohol
- Chronic medical conditions worsened by alcohol:
  - Liver diseases (cirrhosis, hepatitis)
  - Gastrointestinal (GI) diseases (GI bleeding, gastric reflux, ulcer)
  - Cardiovascular diseases (hypertension, heart failure)
  - Metabolic/endocrine diseases (gout, diabetes)
  - Mental disorders (depression, anxiety)
- Alcohol and medication interactions: See Table 9-2.

TABLE 9-2.   Alcohol and Medication Interactions

MEDICATION	RESULT OF CONCURRENT ALCOHOL USE
H$_2$ blockers	Higher BALs
Benzodiazepines, tricyclics, narcotics, barbiturates, antihistamines	↑ sedation
Aspirin, NSAIDs	Prolonged bleeding time; Irritation of gastric lining
Metronidazole, sulfonamides, long-acting hypoglycemics	Nausea and vomiting
Reserpine, nitroglycerin, hydralazine	↑ risk of hypotension
Acetaminophen, isoniazid, phenylbutazone	↑ hepatotoxicity
Antihypertensives, antidiabetics, ulcer drugs, gout medications	Worsen underlying disease

---

KEY FACT

The most common psychiatric disorder in the elderly is major depressive disorder.

KEY FACT

White elderly males have the highest rate of completed suicides.

WARDS TIP

Visual hallucinations early in dementia suggest a diagnosis of neurocognitive disorder due to Lewy body disease. Antipsychotics should be avoided as these patients are sensitive to EPS.

Psychiatric Manifestations of Major Neurocognitive Disorders (Dementia)

Behavioral symptoms are quite common in patients with major neurocognitive disorder, and quite often the source of many psychosocial problems surrounding their care. Agitation and aggression can be distressing and dangerous for caregivers, as well as unsafe for patients. Behavioral disinhibition is fairly common in major neurocognitive disorders and causes patients to act in ways that are quite unlike their typical behaviors (stripping off clothes in public, sexualized behavior, cursing).

- Mood disorders:
    - Difficult to diagnose in a patient with confirmed major neurocognitive disorder.
    - Patients with major neurocognitive disorders may display many symptoms of depression that are merely natural manifestations of their disease.
    - Mood and affect are often poor diagnostic indicators in patients with moderate-to-severe cognitive impairment.
- Aggression:
    - May be provoked by the patient's confusion in the setting of cognitive, memory, and language deficits.
    - May be provoked by hallucinations or delusions.
- Psychosis:
    - Delusions are reported in up to 50% of Alzheimer's patients.
    - Hallucinations (mostly auditory and/or visual) can be seen in at least 25% of patients with a major neurocognitive disorder.
    - If hallucinations do not bother the patient or interfere with caring for the patient, pharmacotherapy is unnecessary.

TREATMENT

Behavioral and environmental treatments for behavioral symptoms are much preferred in the elderly. Pharmacological methods are appropriate in the setting of potentially harmful behaviors, but care must be taken in dosing, duration of treatment, and interactions with other medications.

- Nonpharmacological treatments:
  - Music, art, exercise, and pet therapy.
  - Strict daily schedules to minimize changes in routine.
  - Continual reorientation of patient.
  - Reduce stimuli (quiet living environments).
  - Surround patient with familiar objects (family photos, a favorite quilt, etc.).
- Pharmacological treatments:
  - Antipsychotics:
    - Limited efficacy and ↑ mortality.
    - Try olanzapine (Zyprexa) or quetiapine (Seroquel) in patients with severe symptoms.
    - Can also use short-term haloperidol (Haldol) or risperidone (Risperdal).
  - Anxiolytics:
    - Anxiety symptoms may be due to unrecognized depression and respond well to an SSRI.
    - Reserve benzodiazepines for very short-term, acute episodes and remember to watch for disinhibition (paradoxical agitation).
    - Mood stabilizers: Few studies on their effectiveness in the elderly.

Sleep Disturbance

The incidence of sleep disorders ↑ with aging. Elderly people often report difficulty sleeping, daytime drowsiness, and daytime napping.

- Outside of normal changes associated with aging (see Table 9-3), causes of sleep disturbances may include other medical conditions, drug/alcohol use, social stressors, and medications.
- Patients with movement disorders (Parkinson's disease, progressive supranuclear palsy) have shallow sleep and may be more restless at night because of trouble turning in bed.
- Restless leg movements during sleep, likely due to a dopamine imbalance, are called periodic leg movements (PLMs).
- Nonpharmacological treatment approaches should be tried first (alcohol cessation, ↑ daily structure, elimination of daytime naps, treatment of underlying medical conditions that may be exacerbating sleep problems).

TABLE 9-3. Normal Sleep Changes in Geriatric Patients

Rapid eye movement (REM) sleep	↓ REM latency and ↓ total REM
Non-REM sleep	↑ amounts of stage 1 and 2 sleep, ↓ amounts of stage 3 and 4 sleep (deep sleep)
Sleep efficiency	↓ (frequent nocturnal awakenings)
Amount of total sleep	↓
Sleep cycle	Sleep cycle advances (earlier to bed, earlier to rise)

- Sedative-hypnotic drugs are more likely to cause side effects when used by the elderly (memory impairment, ataxia, paradoxical excitement, and rebound insomnia).
- If sedative-hypnotics must be prescribed, medications such as trazodone are safer than the more sedating benzodiazepines, but be careful of orthostasis.

Other Issues

RESTRAINTS

- In nonemergency situations, restraints should be used as a last resort and the patient should be reassessed at regular intervals.
- Patient safety, health, and well-being should be the most important concern in the matter of restraint use.

MEDICATIONS

- Many older people are on multiple medications.
- They suffer from more side effects because of ↓ lean body mass and impaired liver and kidney function.
- When confronted with a new symptom in an elderly patient on multiple medications, always try to remove a medication before adding one.

ELDER ABUSE

- Types: Physical abuse, psychological abuse (threats, insults, etc.), neglect (withholding of care), exploitation (misuse of finances), and rarely sexual abuse.
- Approximately 10% of all people >65 years old; underreported by victims.
- Perpetrator is usually a caregiver (spouse or adult child) who lives with the victim.

NURSING HOMES

- Provide care and rehabilitation for chronically ill and impaired patients as well as for patients who are in need of short-term care before returning to their prior living arrangements.
- The majority of patients stay permanently, and fewer than half are discharged after only a short period of time.

CHAPTER 10

PSYCHIATRIC DISORDERS IN CHILDREN

Psychiatric Examination of a Child	122
SOURCES OF INFORMATION	122
METHODS OF GATHERING INFORMATION	122
Intellectual Disability	122
DIAGNOSIS AND DSM-5 CRITERIA	122
EPIDEMIOLOGY	122
ETIOLOGY	123
Global Developmental Delay	123
Specific Learning Disorder	123
DIAGNOSIS AND DSM-5 CRITERIA	123
EPIDEMIOLOGY	124
ETIOLOGY	124
COMORBIDITY	124
TREATMENT	124
Communication Disorders	124
TREATMENT	124
Attention Deficit/Hyperactivity Disorder (ADHD)	125
DIAGNOSIS AND DSM-5 CRITERIA	125
EPIDEMIOLOGY	126
ETIOLOGY	126
COURSE/PROGNOSIS	126
TREATMENT	126
Autism Spectrum Disorder (ASD)	126
DIAGNOSIS AND DSM-5 CRITERIA	127
EPIDEMIOLOGY	127
ETIOLOGY	127
PROGNOSIS AND TREATMENT	127
Tic Disorders	128
TOURETTE'S DISORDER	128
Disruptive and Conduct Disorders	129
OPPOSITIONAL DEFIANT DISORDER (ODD)	129
CONDUCT DISORDER	129
Elimination Disorders	130
DSM-5 DIAGNOSIS	130
EPIDEMIOLOGY	131
ETIOLOGY	131
TREATMENT	131
Child Abuse	131
PHYSICAL ABUSE	132
SEXUAL ABUSE	132
PSYCHOLOGICAL ABUSE	132
NEGLECT	132
TREATMENT	132
SEQUELAE	132

Psychiatric Examination of a Child

SOURCES OF INFORMATION

Gather and integrate collateral information from multiple sources to obtain as accurate a clinical picture as possible: primary caregivers, teachers, pediatricians, and the child welfare system (if relevant).

METHODS OF GATHERING INFORMATION

Determine the child's **developmental stage** and tailor the interview appropriately.

- **Play therapy:** Utilizes the child's symbolic *play, storytelling,* or *drawing as a forum for expression of emotions and experiences.*
- **Classroom observation:** A window into the child's functioning in school.
- **Formal neuropsychological testing:** Quantitatively assesses a child's strengths and weaknesses by examination of cognitive profile: intelligence quotient (IQ); language and visual-motor skills; memory, attention, and organizational abilities.
- **Kaufman Assessment Battery for Children (K-ABC):** Intelligence test comparing intellectual capacity with acquired knowledge of patients between 2 and 12 years old.
- **Wechsler Intelligence Scale for Children-Revised (WISC-R):** Assesses verbal, performance, and full-scale IQ of patients between 6 and 16 years old.

Intellectual Disability

Intellectual disability (ID, intellectual developmental disorder) replaces the term mental retardation (MR) as per US law (Rosa's Law), with the intention of decreasing stigmatization. ID is characterized by **severely impaired cognitive** and adaptive/**social functioning.** Severity level is currently based on adaptive functioning, indicating degree of support required. A single IQ score does not adequately capture this and is no longer used solely to determine ID severity.

DIAGNOSIS AND DSM-5 CRITERIA

- **Deficits in intellectual functioning,** such as reasoning, problem solving, planning, abstract thinking, judgment, and learning
- **Deficits in adaptive functioning,** such as communication, social participation, and independent living
- Deficits affect multiple domains: conceptual, practical, and social
- Onset during the developmental period
- Intellectual deficits confirmed by clinical assessment and standardized intelligence testing (scores at least 2 standard deviations below the population mean)
- Adaptive functioning deficits require **ongoing support for activities of daily life**
- Severity levels: mild, moderate, severe, profound

EPIDEMIOLOGY

- Overall: 1% of population
- Severe ID: 6/1000

TABLE 10-1.   Causes of Mental Retardation

Cause	Examples
Genetic	**Down syndrome:** Trisomy 21 (1/700 live births)
	Fragile X syndrome: Involves mutation of X chromosome, second most common cause of intellectual disability, M > F
	Others: Phenylketonuria, familial mental retardation, Prader-Willi syndrome, Williams syndrome, Angelman syndrome, tuberous sclerosis
Prenatal	Infection and toxins (**TORCH**):
	■ **T**oxoplasmosis
	■ **O**ther (syphilis, AIDS, alcohol/illicit drugs)
	■ **R**ubella (German measles)
	■ **C**ytomegalovirus (CMV)
	■ **H**erpes simplex
Perinatal	Anoxia, prematurity, birth trauma, meningitis, hyperbilirubinemia
Postnatal	Hypothyroidism, malnutrition, toxin exposure, trauma, psychosocial causes

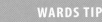

WARDS TIP

Characteristic physical features of Genetic Syndromes
- Down syndrome: epicanthic folds, flat nasal bridge, and palmar crease
- Fragile X syndrome: macrocephaly, joint hyperlaxity, and macroorchidism in postpubertal males
- Prader–Willi syndrome: obese, small stature, and almond-shaped eyes

KEY FACT

Fragile X Syndrome Facts and Stats
- Most common inherited form of ID
- 2nd most common cause of ID
- Due to *FMR*-1 gene mutation
- Males > Females

KEY FACT

Down Syndrome Facts and Stats
- 1/700 live births
- Most common chromosomal disorder
- Trisomy 21 = 3 copies of chromosome 21

KEY FACT

Fetal Alcohol Exposure Facts
- Fetal Alcohol Syndrome (FAS) = Leading *preventable* cause of birth defects and ID

Three features of FAS
1. Growth retardation
2. CNS involvement (structural, neurologic, functional)
3. Facial dysmorphology (smooth philtrum, short palpebral fissures, thin vermillion border)
   - Fetal alcohol exposure may cause a range of developmental disabilities, including ID

ETIOLOGY

Fifty percent of ID has no identifiable cause. Other causes include genetic, prenatal, perinatal, and postnatal conditions (see Table 10-1).

Global Developmental Delay

- Failure to meet expected developmental milestones in several areas of intellectual functioning
- Diagnosis reserved for patients <5 years old when severity level cannot be reliably assessed via standardized testing. Patients will need to be reevaluated to clarify the diagnosis at a later time.

Specific Learning Disorder

Characterized by delayed cognitive development in a particular academic domain. Challenges with reading, writing, and arithmetic often co-occur. Specific learning disorder frequently occurs with ADHD, which can worsen the prognosis.

DIAGNOSIS AND DSM-5 CRITERIA

- Significantly impaired academic skills which are below expected for the chronological age and interfere with schooling, occupation, or activities of daily living (ADLs)
- Begins during school-age but may become more impairing as demands increase

- Affected areas: reading (e.g., dyslexia), writing, or arithmetic (e.g., dyscalculia)
- Not better accounted for by intellectual disabilities, visual/auditory deficits, language barriers, or subpar education

EPIDEMIOLOGY

- Prevalence in school age children: 5–15%
- Males > females affected

ETIOLOGY

- Environmental factors: ↑ risk with prematurity, very low birth weight, prenatal nicotine use
- Genetic factors: ↑ risk in first-degree relatives of affected individuals

COMORBIDITY

- Commonly co-occurs with other neurodevelopmental disorders, such as ADHD, communication disorders, developmental coordination disorder, autistic spectrum disorder
- Also comorbid with other mental disorders, including anxiety, depressive, and bipolar disorders

TREATMENT

- Systematic, individualized education tailored to child's specific needs
- Behavioral techniques may be used to improve learning skills

Communication Disorders

Encompass impaired speech, language or social communication that are below those expected for chronological age, begin in the early developmental period, and lead to academic or adaptive issues

- Language disorder—difficulty acquiring and using language due to expressive and/or receptive impairment (e.g., reduced vocabulary, limited sentence structure, impairments in discourse). ↑ risk in families of affected individuals
- Speech sound disorder (Phonological disorder)—difficulty producing articulate, intelligible speech
- Childhood-onset fluency disorder (Stuttering)—dysfluency and speech motor production issues. ↑ risk of stuttering in first-degree relatives of affected individuals
- Social (Pragmatic) communication disorder—challenges with the **social use of verbal and nonverbal communication. If restricted/repetitive behaviors, activities, or interests also present → diagnose autism spectrum disorder (ASD).** ↑ risk with family history of communication disorders, ASD, or specific learning disorder.

TREATMENT

- Speech and language therapy, family counseling
- Tailor education to meet the individual's needs

An 8-year-old girl, Matty Ryan, is referred for evaluation because of academic and behavior problems at school and home for the last year. Her mother reports that Matty is constantly on the move, never sits still, and appears to be "driven by a motor." Mrs. Ryan complains that Matty does not pay attention when she is told to do something or "says she forgets."

Matty's teacher reports that she does not follow directions. She has trouble waiting her turn and often blurts out answers during class. While Matty also makes a lot of careless mistakes on homework she seems to comprehend the material.

What is the most likely diagnosis?

Matty Ryan has classic symptoms of attention deficit/hyperactivity disorder (ADHD), with both inattention and hyperactivity in two different settings (home and school).

What treatment is indicated?

Stimulant medications are considered to be the first-line treatment for ADHD.

Attention Deficit/Hyperactivity Disorder (ADHD)

ADHD is characterized by persistent **inattention**, **hyperactivity**, and **impulsivity inconsistent** with the patient's **developmental stage**. There are three subcategories of ADHD: predominantly inattentive type, predominantly hyperactive/impulsive type, and combined type.

DIAGNOSIS AND DSM-5 CRITERIA

- Two symptom domains: inattentiveness and hyperactivity/impulsivity
- At least **six inattentive symptoms**
  - Fails to give close attention to details or makes careless mistakes.
  - Has difficulty sustaining attention.
  - Does not appear to listen.
  - Struggles to follow through on instructions.
  - Has difficulty with organization.
  - Avoids or dislikes tasks requiring a lot of thinking.
  - Loses things.
  - Is easily distracted.
  - Is forgetful in daily activities.

and/or

- At least **six hyperactivity/impulsivity symptoms**
  - Fidgets with hands or feet or squirms in chair.
  - Has difficulty remaining seated.
  - Runs about or climbs excessively in childhood; extreme restlessness in adults.
  - Difficulty engaging in activities quietly.
  - Acts as if driven by a motor; may be an internal sensation in adults.

- - Talks excessively.
  - Blurts out answers before questions have been completed.
  - Difficulty waiting or taking turns.
  - Interrupts or intrudes upon others.
- Symptoms >6 months and present in two or more settings (e.g., home, school, work)
- Symptoms interfere with or reduce quality of social/academic/occupational functioning
- Onset **prior to age 12, but** can be diagnosed retrospectively in adulthood
- Symptoms not due to another mental disorder

EPIDEMIOLOGY

- Prevalence: 5% of children and 2.5% of adults
- Males:females with 2:1 ratio

Females present more often with inattentive symptoms.

ETIOLOGY

The etiology of ADHD is multifactorial and may include:

- Genetic factors: ↑ rate in first-degree relatives of affected individuals
- Environmental factors: low birth weight, smoking during pregnancy, childhood abuse/neglect, neurotoxin/alcohol exposure

COURSE/PROGNOSIS

- Stable through adolescence
- Many continue to have symptoms as adults (inattentive > hyperactive)
- High incidence of comorbid oppositional defiant disorder, conduct disorder (CD), and specific learning disorder

TREATMENT

Multimodal treatment plan: medications are the most effective treatment for decreasing core symptoms, but should be used in conjunction with educational and behavioral interventions.

- Pharmacological treatments:
  - First-line: Stimulants—methylphenidate compounds, dextroamphetamine, and mixed amphetamine salts
  - Second-line choice: atomoxetine, a norepinephrine reuptake inhibitor
  - Alpha-2 agonists (e.g., clonidine, **guanfacine**) can be used instead of or as adjunctive therapy to stimulants
- Nonpharmacological treatments:
  - Behavior modification techniques and social skills training
  - Educational interventions (i.e., classroom modifications)
  - Parent psychoeducation

KEY FACT

Stimulants are first-line therapy in ADHD.

Autism Spectrum Disorder (ASD)

ASD is characterized by impairments in **social communication/interaction and restrictive, repetitive behaviors/interests**. This disorder encompasses the spectrum of symptomatology formerly diagnosed as autism, Asperger's disorder, childhood disintegrative disorder, and pervasive developmental disorder.

DIAGNOSIS AND DSM-5 CRITERIA

- **Problems with social interaction and communication:**
  - impaired social/emotional reciprocity (e.g., inability to hold conversations)
  - deficits in nonverbal communication skills (e.g., decreased eye contact)
  - interpersonal/relational challenges (e.g., lack of interest in peers)
- **Restricted, repetitive patterns of behavior, interests, and activities:**
  - intense, peculiar interests (e.g., preoccupation with unusual objects)
  - inflexible adherence to rituals (e.g., rigid thought patterns)
  - stereotyped, repetitive motor mannerisms (e.g., hand flapping)
  - hyper/hyporeactivity to sensory input (e.g., hypersensitive to particular textures)
- Abnormalities in functioning begin in the early developmental period.
- Not better accounted for by ID or global developmental delay. When ID and ASD co-occur, social communication is below expectation based on developmental level.
- Causes significant social or occupational impairment.

EPIDEMIOLOGY

- Recent ↑ in prevalence: 1% of population
  Could be related to expansion of diagnostic classification and/or ↑ awareness/recognition
- 4:1 ratio of diagnosis in males:females
- Symptoms typically recognized between 12 and 24 months old, but varies based on severity

ETIOLOGY

Etiology of ASD is multifactorial:

- Prenatal neurological insults (e.g., infections, drugs), advanced paternal age, low birth weight
- 15% of ASD cases are associated with a known genetic mutation
- Fragile X syndrome = most common known single gene cause of ASD
- Other genetic causes of ASD: Down's syndrome, Rett syndrome, tuberous sclerosis
- High comorbidity with ID
- Association with epilepsy

PROGNOSIS AND TREATMENT

ASD is a chronic condition. The prognosis is variable, but the two most important predictors of adult outcome are level of intellectual functioning and language impairment. Only a minority of patients is able to live and work independently in adulthood. There is no cure for autism, but various treatments are used to help manage symptoms and improve basic social, communicative, and cognitive skills:

- Early intervention
- Remedial education
- Behavioral therapy
- Psychoeducation
- Low dose atypical antipsychotic medications (e.g., risperidone, aripiprazole) may help reduce disruptive behavior, aggression, and irritability.

WARDS TIP

Red flag for ASD: rapid deterioration of social and/or language skills during first 2 years of life.

Complete an appropriate workup, such as auditory testing, prior to diagnosing ASD.

If skills are lost after age 2 or more expansive losses occur (e.g., self-care, motor skills), an extensive medical workup needs to be initiated.

WARDS TIP

Assess for a potential cause of pain/discomfort if a nonverbal ASD patient presents with new onset aggression or self-injurious behavior.

Tic Disorders

TOURETTE'S DISORDER

Tics are defined as sudden, rapid, repetitive, stereotyped movements or vocalizations. Although experienced as involuntary, patients can learn to temporarily suppress tics. Prior to the tic, patients may feel a premonitory urge (somatic sensation), with subsequent tension release after the tic. Anxiety, excitement, and fatigue can be aggravating factors for tics.

Tourette's disorder is the most severe of the tic disorders. It is characterized by **multiple motor tics and at least one vocal tic lasting for at least 1 year.** Vocal tics may appear many years after the motor tics, and they may wax and wane in frequency. The most common **motor tics** involve the face and head, such as eye blinking and throat clearing.

Examples of **vocal tics**:

- *Coprolalia*—utterance of obscene, taboo words as an abrupt, sharp bark or grunt
- *Echolalia*—repeating others' words

Diagnosis and DSM-5 Criteria

- Multiple motor and ≥ 1 vocal tics present (not required to occur concurrently) for >1 year since onset of first tic
- Onset prior to age 18 years
- Not caused by a substance (e.g., cocaine) or another medical condition (e.g., Huntington's disease)

Epidemiology

- Transient tic behaviors: common in children
- Tourette's disorder: 3 per 1000 school-age children
- Prevalence: boys > girls

Etiology

- Genetic factors: $>55\%$ concordance rate in monozygotic twins
- Pre/perinatal factors: older paternal age, obstetrical complications, maternal smoking, and low birth weight
- Psychological factors: symptom exacerbations with stressful life events

Course/prognosis

- Onset typically occurs between 4 and 6 years, with the peak severity between ages 10 and 12
- Tics wax and wane and change in type
- Symptoms tend to decrease in adolescence and significantly diminish in adulthood
- High comorbidity with obsessive-compulsive disorder and ADHD

Treatment

- Psychoeducation
- **Behavioral interventions**—habit reversal therapy
- Medications—utilize only if tics become impairing. Due to the fluctuating course of the disorder, it can be difficult to determine medication efficacy.

WARDS TIP

Tic disorders are one of the few psychiatric disorders in which diagnostic criteria do not require symptoms to cause significant distress.

- **Alpha-2 agonists: guanfacine (first choice)**, clonidine (more sedating)
- In severe cases, can consider treatment with atypical (e.g., risperidone) or typical antipsychotics (e.g., pimozide)

Other tic disorders include **PERSISTENT (CHRONIC) MOTOR OR VOCAL TIC DISORDER** (Single or multiple motor or vocal tics [but not both] that have never met criteria for Tourette's) and **PROVISIONAL TIC DISORDER** (Single or multiple motor and/or vocal tics <1 year that have never met criteria for Tourette's).

Disruptive and Conduct Disorders

These disorders involve **problematic interactions** or **inflicting harm** on others. While disruptive behaviors may appear within the scope of normal development, they become pathologic when the **frequency, pervasiveness, and severity impair functioning of the individual or of others.**

OPPOSITIONAL DEFIANT DISORDER (ODD)

A maladaptive pattern of **irritability/anger, defiance, or vindictiveness**, which causes dysfunction, or **distress in the patient or those affected**. These interpersonal issues involve at least one non-sibling.

Diagnosis and DSM-5 Criteria

Characterized by at least four symptoms present for ≥6 months (with at least one individual who is not a sibling):

- **Anger/Irritable Mood**—loses temper; touchy/easily annoyed; often angry/resentful
- **Argumentative/Defiant Behavior**—breaks rules; argues with authority figures; deliberately annoys others; blames others
- **Vindictiveness**—spiteful at least 2× in past 6 months
- Disturbance is associated with distress in the individual or others, or it impacts negatively on functioning
- Behaviors do not occur exclusively during another mental disorder

Epidemiology

- Prevalence: Approximately 3%
- Onset usually during preschool years: seen more often in boys before adolescence
- ↑ incidence of comorbid substance use and ADHD
- Although ODD often precedes CD, most do not develop CD.

Treatment

- **Behavior modification**, conflict management training, and improving problem-solving skills.
- Parent Management Training (PMT) can help with setting limits and enforcing consistent rules.
- Medications are used to treat comorbid conditions, such as ADHD.

CONDUCT DISORDER

CD includes the **most serious disruptive behaviors, which violate the rights of other humans and animals**. These individuals inflict cruelty and harm

WARDS TIP

If a child has no difficulties getting along with peers but will not comply with rules from parents or teachers, consider the diagnosis of *oppositional defiant disorder.*

KEY FACT

Unlike conduct disorder, ODD does *not* involve physical aggression or violating others' basic rights.

KEY FACT

Cruelty to animals may be indicative of Conduct disorder.

through **physical and sexual violence**. They may **lack remorse** for committing crimes or **lack empathy** for their victims.

Diagnosis and DSM-5 Criteria

A pattern of **recurrently violating the basic rights of others or societal norms**, with at least three behaviors exhibited over the last year and at least one occurring within the past 6 months.

- **Aggression to people and animals:** Bullies/threatens/intimidates others; initiates physical fights; uses weapon; physically cruel to people; physically cruel to animals; stolen items while confronting victim; forced someone into sexual activity.
- **Destruction of property:** Engaged in fire setting; destroyed property by other means.
- **Deceitfulness or Theft:** Broken into a home/building/car; lied to obtain goods/favors; stolen items without confronting a victim.
- **Serious violations of rules:** Stays out late at night before 13 years old; runs away from home overnight at least twice; often truant from school before 13 years old

Epidemiology

- Lifetime prevalence: 9%
- More common in males
- High incidence of comorbid ADHD and ODD
- Associated with antisocial personality disorder

Treatment

- A multimodal treatment approach with **behavior modification**, family, and community involvement.
- PMT can help parents with limit setting and enforcing consistent rules.
- Medications can be used to target comorbid symptoms and aggression (e.g., SSRIs, guanfacine, propranolol, mood stabilizers, antipsychotics).

Elimination Disorders

Characterized by **developmentally inappropriate elimination of urine or feces**. Though typically involuntary, this may be intentional. The course may be *primary* (never established continence) or *secondary* (continence achieved for a period and then lost). Incontinence can cause significant distress or impair social or other areas of functioning.

DSM-5 DIAGNOSIS

Enuresis:

- **Recurrent urination into clothes or bed-wetting**
- Occurs 2×/week for ≥3 consecutive months or results in clinical distress or marked impairment
- ≥5 years old developmentally
- Can occur **during sleep (nocturnal), waking hours (diurnal), or both**
- Not due to a substance (e.g., diuretic) or another medical condition (e.g., urinary tract infection, neurogenic bladder, diabetes)

Encopresis:

- **Recurrent defecation into inappropriate places (e.g., clothes, floor)**
- Occurs ≥1×/month for ≥3 months

KEY FACT

Male versus Female Misconduct

Males: Higher risk of fighting, stealing, fire-setting, and vandalism

Females: Higher risk of lying, running away, prostitution, and substance use

- ≥4 years old developmentally
- Not due to a substance (e.g., laxatives) or another medical condition (e.g., hypothyroidism, anal fissure, spina bifida) except via a constipation-related mechanism

EPIDEMIOLOGY

- Prevalence of enuresis ↓ with age:
  - 5–10% of 5 year olds; 3–5% of 10 year olds; 1% of >15 years old
  - Nocturnal enuresis more common in boys; diurnal enuresis more common in girls
- Prevalence of encopresis: 1% of 5-year-old children; boys > girls

ETIOLOGY

- Genetic predisposition for nocturnal enuresis:
  - About 4× ↑ risk if maternal urinary incontinence
  - About 10× ↑ risk if paternal urinary incontinence
- Psychosocial stressors may contribute to secondary incontinence
- Encopresis: often related to constipation/impaction with overflow incontinence

TREATMENT

- Take into account the high spontaneous remission rates.
- **Psychoeducation** is key for children and their primary caregivers.
- Only treat if symptoms are distressing and impairing. Engage the patient as an active participant in the treatment plan. Encourage investment in a waterproof mattress.
- PMT for managing intentional elimination.
- **Enuresis treatment:**
  - Limit fluid intake and caffeine at night.
  - Behavioral program with monitoring and reward system, "bladder training" exercises, or **urine alarm** (upgrade from the **"bell and pad" method**)
  - Pharmacology can be used if the above methods are ineffective or for diurnal enuresis.
    - **Desmopressin (DDAVP)**, an antidiuretic hormone analogue, is the **first-line medication**.
    - **Imipramine**, a tricyclic antidepressant, can be used at low doses for refractory cases but has less tolerable side effects.
- **Encopresis without constipation:** comprehensive behavioral program ("bowel retraining") for appropriate elimination
- **Encopresis due to constipation:** initial bowel cleaning followed by stool softeners, high-fiber diet, and toileting routine in conjunction with a behavioral program

WARDS TIP

The majority of enuresis cases spontaneously remit (5–10% per year) by adolescence.

Child Abuse

Child abuse encompasses physical abuse, sexual abuse, emotional abuse, and neglect. **Toxic stress** may result when children **endure prolonged, severe trauma and adversity** without the buffer of supportive caregivers. This can disrupt a child's development and lead to a spectrum of pathologic sequelae.

- About **1 million** cases of **child maltreatment** in the United States
- Up to 2500 deaths/year caused by abuse in the United States

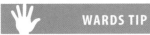

WARDS TIP

Red flags for physical abuse: Delayed medical care for injury, inconsistent explanation of injury, multiple injuries in various stages of healing, spiral bone fractures, bruising patterns consistent with hand/belt, cigarette burns, and head injuries.

WARDS TIP

Red flags for sexual abuse: Sexually transmitted diseases, recurrent urinary tract infections, prepubertal vaginal bleeding, pregnancy, or trauma/bruising/inflammation of genitals or anus. Developmentally inappropriate sexual knowledge/behaviors should also raise suspicion.

WARDS TIP

If a child reports sexual abuse, it should be taken seriously as it is rarely unfounded.

KEY FACT

Alcohol is the most common drug of abuse by adolescents, followed by cannabis.

WARDS TIP

Doctors are *mandated reporters*, thus legally required to report all cases of suspected child abuse to the appropriate social service agencies.

These numbers may be an underestimation as many cases go undetected and unreported.

PHYSICAL ABUSE

- Any act that results in nonaccidental injury and may be the result of severe corporal punishment committed by an individual with responsibility for the child.
- Physical exam and x-rays may demonstrate multiple, concerning injuries not consistent with child's developmental age.
- Most common perpetrator is first-degree caregiver (e.g., parent, guardian, mother's boyfriend).

SEXUAL ABUSE

- Any sexual act involving a child intended to provide sexual gratification to an individual who has responsibility for the child.
- Sexual abuse is the most invasive form of abuse and results in detrimental lifetime effects on victim.
- Approximately 25% of girls and 9% of boys are exposed to *sexual* abuse.
- The victim of sexual abuse is typically female (*although boys are less likely to report*). The perpetrator is usually male and known to the victim.
- Children are most at risk of sexual abuse during preadolescence.

PSYCHOLOGICAL ABUSE

- Nonaccidental verbal or symbolic acts that result in psychological damage

NEGLECT

- Failure to provide a child with adequate food, shelter, supervision, medical care, education, and/or affection
- Victims of neglect may exhibit poor hygiene, malnutrition, stunted growth, developmental delay, and failure to thrive
- Severe deprivation can result in death, particularly in infants
- Neglect accounts for the majority of cases reported to child protection services

TREATMENT

- Early intervention can potentially mitigate the negative sequelae and facilitate recovery.

SEQUELAE

- ↑ risk of developing posttraumatic stress disorder, anxiety disorders, depressive disorders, dissociative disorders, self-destructive behaviors, and substance use disorders
- ↑ risk of continuing abuse cycle with their own children

CHAPTER 11

DISSOCIATIVE DISORDERS

Dissociative Amnesia   134

    DIAGNOSIS AND DSM-5 CRITERIA   134

    EPIDEMIOLOGY/ETIOLOGY   134

    TREATMENT   134

Depersonalization/Derealization Disorder   135

    DIAGNOSIS AND DSM-5 CRITERIA   135

    EPIDEMIOLOGY/ETIOLOGY   135

    COURSE AND PROGNOSIS   135

    TREATMENT   135

Dissociative Identity Disorder (Multiple Personality Disorder)   136

    DIAGNOSIS AND DSM-5 CRITERIA   136

    EPIDEMIOLOGY/ETIOLOGY   136

    COURSE AND PROGNOSIS   136

    TREATMENT   136

Other Specified Dissociative Disorder   136

    DSM-5 EXAMPLES   137

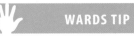
WARDS TIP

Dissociative responses can occur during stressful and traumatic events.

KEY FACT

Although dissociative fugue is now considered a subtype of dissociative amnesia disorder, it more commonly occurs in dissociative identity disorder.

KEY FACT

Dissociative amnesia refers to disruption in the continuity of an individual's memory. Patients with dissociative amnesia report gaps in the recollection of particular events, usually traumatic ones.

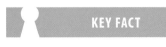
WARDS TIP

Patients suffering from dissociative amnesia can experience periods of flashbacks, nightmares, or behavioral reenactments of their trauma.

KEY FACT

Abreaction is the strong emotional reaction patients may experience when retrieving traumatic memories.

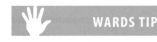
WARDS TIP

Fu*gue*: Remember as a *fugitive* who runs away and forms a new identity.

Dissociation can be understood as a **disruption in the integrated sense of self**. This may involve **lapses in autobiographical memory** (*amnesia*) and **feelings of detachment from one's self** (*depersonalization*) or from one's surroundings (*derealization*). These symptoms often develop in the context or aftermath of **significant trauma**, particularly **during childhood**. Dissociation may initially help buffer the impact of a trauma, but can become pathological and maladaptive.

Dissociative Amnesia

These patients are unable to remember important personal information or history, often **traumatic** in nature. **Procedural memory is preserved**, distinguishing dissociative amnesia from other conditions resulting in memory loss (e.g., major neurocognitive disorders or dementias). The unrecalled autobiographical information has been stored in memory and thus is potentially retrievable. Dissociative amnesia rarely generalizes to encompass complete memory loss. There is a significant incidence of comorbid major depressive disorder or persistent depressive disorder (dysthymia) and an **increased risk for suicide**—particularly as amnesia resolves and the overwhelming memories return.

DIAGNOSIS AND DSM-5 CRITERIA

- An inability to recall important autobiographical information, usually involving a traumatic or stressful event, that is inconsistent with ordinary forgetfulness.
- May present with *dissociative fugue* symptoms: **sudden, unexpected travel away from home**, accompanied by amnesia for identity or other autobiographical information.
- Not due to the physiological effects of a substance or another medical/psychiatric/neurological disorder (including traumatic brain injury).
- Symptoms cause significant distress or impairment in daily functioning.

EPIDEMIOLOGY/ETIOLOGY

- Lifetime prevalence is 6–7%
- More common in women than men
- Single or repeated traumas often occur prior to amnesia

TREATMENT

- Important to establish the patient's safety.
- Removal from the traumatic situation often will bring back the memories.
- Psychotherapy (e.g., supportive, CBT, hypnosis) is the mainstay of treatment.
- No medications have demonstrated efficacy in dissociative amnesia.

A 19-year-old male is found 3 days after being reported missing. He was wandering around miles away from his home. When questioned, he could not recall his full name or where he was from. His wallet reveals an ID with the name, Charles Henderson, from Edmond, Oklahoma. His family reports that he recently returned home from the military.

Likely diagnosis? Dissociative amnesia with dissociative fugue

Depersonalization/Derealization Disorder

Characterized by repeated experiences of **detachment from one's self or surroundings**. Patients may feel as though they are observing themselves from a distance or have an **"out-of-body"** experience (*depersonalization*). They may experience the world around them as though they were **in a dream or movie** (*derealization*).

DIAGNOSIS AND DSM-5 CRITERIA

- Persistent or recurrent experiences of one or both:
  - Depersonalization—Experiences of unreality or detachment from one's body, thoughts, feelings, or actions
  - Derealization—Experiences of unreality or detachment from one's surroundings
- Reality testing remains intact during episode
- The symptoms cause significant distress or social/occupational impairment
- Not accounted for by a substance (e.g., drug of abuse, medication), another medical condition, or another mental disorder

EPIDEMIOLOGY/ETIOLOGY

- Lifetime prevalence is 2%.
- Gender ratio 1:1.
- Mean age of onset about 16 years old.
- ↑ incidence of comorbid anxiety disorders and major depression.
- Severe stress or traumas are predisposing factors.

COURSE AND PROGNOSIS

Often persistent but may wax and wane.

TREATMENT

- Psychodynamic, cognitive-behavioral, hypnotherapy, and supportive therapies may be helpful.
- Lack of evidence for use of medications to treat depersonalization/derealization disorder.

KEY FACT

Transient experiences of depersonalization or derealization commonly occur in many individuals during times of stress.

A 21-year-old woman is brought by her boyfriend to the clinic for evaluation. He reports concern that she "is having memory issues and acting like somebody else completely." The boyfriend reports that the patient recently went home for the holidays and "had to deal with her abusive, alcoholic father. She hasn't seemed the same since she got back."

The patient seems oblivious to his concerns and denies any complaints. In fact, she insists on being called by another name and denies knowing her boyfriend.

Most likely diagnosis? Dissociative Identity Disorder (DID)

Dissociative Identity Disorder (Multiple Personality Disorder)

Dissociative identity disorder (DID) is characterized by the presence of **more than one distinct personality state** as a result of a fragmented sense of self. DID encompasses features of the other dissociative disorders, such as **amnesia, depersonalization**, and **derealization**. DID predominantly develops in **victims of significant and chronic/childhood trauma**. Patients diagnosed with DID often cope with posttraumatic stress disorder, depression, and suicidality.

DIAGNOSIS AND DSM-5 CRITERIA

- **Disruption of identity** manifested **as two or more distinct personality states** dominating at different times. These symptoms may be observed by others or self-reported.
- **Extensive memory lapses** in autobiographical information, daily occurrences, and/or traumatic events.
- Not due to effects of a substance (drug or medication) or another medical condition.
- The condition causes significant distress or impairment in social/occupational functioning.

EPIDEMIOLOGY/ETIOLOGY

- Rare (<1%), but prevalence higher in women than men.
- Childhood physical/sexual abuse or neglect present in 90% of patients with DID.
- May manifest at any age, but some symptoms are usually present in childhood.
- High incidence of comorbid PTSD, major depression, eating disorders, borderline personality disorder, and substance use disorders.
- >70% of patients attempt suicide, often with frequent attempts and self-mutilation.

COURSE AND PROGNOSIS

- Course is fluctuating but chronic.
- Worst prognosis of all dissociative disorders.

TREATMENT

- Psychotherapy is the standard treatment. The focus should be on safety, stabilization, and symptom reduction, working directly with traumatic memories, and identity integration.
- Pharmacotherapy: SSRIs to target comorbid depressive and/or PTSD symptoms (especially hyperarousal). Prazosin may help target nightmares and naltrexone may help reduce self-mutilation.

Other Specified Dissociative Disorder

Characterized by symptoms of dissociation that cause significant distress or impairment of functioning, but do not meet the full criteria for a specific dissociative disorder.

WARDS TIP

Symptoms of multiple personality disorder may be similar to those seen in borderline personality disorder or psychotic disorders.

DSM-5 EXAMPLES

- Identity disturbance due to prolonged and intense coercive persuasion (e.g., brainwashing, torture, cults)
- Chronic and recurrent syndromes of mixed dissociative symptoms (without dissociative amnesia)
- Dissociative trance (an acute narrowing or loss of awareness of surroundings manifesting as unresponsiveness, potentially with minor stereotyped behaviors; it is not part of a cultural or religious practice)
- Acute dissociative reactions to stressful events (lasting hours/days → 1 month)

CHAPTER 12

SOMATIC SYMPTOM AND FACTITIOUS DISORDERS

Somatic Symptom Disorder	140
DIAGNOSIS AND DSM-5 CRITERIA	141
EPIDEMIOLOGY	141
TREATMENT AND PROGNOSIS	141
Conversion Disorder (Functional Neurological Symptom Disorder)	141
DIAGNOSIS AND DSM-5 CRITERIA	141
EPIDEMIOLOGY	141
TREATMENT AND PROGNOSIS	142
Illness Anxiety Disorder	142
DIAGNOSIS AND DSM-5 CRITERIA	142
EPIDEMIOLOGY	142
TREATMENT	142
PROGNOSIS	142
Psychological Factors Affecting Other Medical Conditions	142
DIAGNOSIS AND DSM-5 CRITERIA	143
EPIDEMIOLOGY	143
TREATMENT AND PROGNOSIS	143
Factitious Disorder	143
DIAGNOSIS AND DSM-5 CRITERIA	143
EPIDEMIOLOGY	143
TREATMENT AND PROGNOSIS	144
Malingering	144
PRESENTATION	144
EPIDEMIOLOGY	144
Review of Distinguishing Features	144

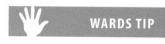

KEY FACT

Malingering is the *conscious* feigning of symptoms in order to avoid jail, court, or obtain housing or compensation.

WARDS TIP

When treating a patient with a somatic symptom disorder, it is important to work closely with the patient's primary care physician.

Patients with somatic symptom disorders present with prominent somatic symptoms associated with significant distress or impairment in social, occupational, or other areas of functioning. While these patients may or may not have an associated medical condition, their focus is on their distressing somatic symptoms as well as their thoughts, feelings, and behaviors in response to these symptoms.

- Types of somatic symptom and related disorders include:
  - Somatic symptom disorder
  - Conversion disorder (functional neurological symptom disorder)
  - Illness anxiety disorder
  - Psychological factors affecting other medical conditions
  - Factious disorder
  - Other specified somatic symptom and related disorder
  - Unspecified somatic symptom and related disorder

Somatic symptom disorders are likely more common in women.

> Ms. Thomas is a 31-year-old woman who was referred to a psychiatrist by her gynecologist after undergoing multiple exploratory surgeries for abdominal pain and gynecologic concerns with no definitive findings. The patient reports that she has had extensive medical problems dating back to adolescence. She reports periods of extreme abdominal pain, vomiting, diarrhea, and possible food intolerances. The obstetrician is her fourth provider because "my other doctors were not able to help me." Ms. Thomas reports fear that her current physician will also fail to relieve her distress. She was reluctant to see a psychiatrist and did so only after her obstetrician agreed to follow her after her psychiatric appointment.
>
> Ms. Thomas states that her problems worsened in college, which was the first time she underwent surgery. She reports that due to her health problems and severe lack of energy, it took her 5½ years to graduate from college. She did better for a year or two after college but then had a return of symptoms. She reports recently feeling very lonely and isolated because she has not been able to find a boyfriend who can tolerate her frequent illnesses. She also reports that physical intimacy is difficult for her because she finds sex painful. Additionally, she is concerned that she might lose her job due to the number of days she has missed from work due to her abdominal pain, fatigue, and weakness.
>
> ### What is the diagnosis?
>
> Somatic symptom disorder. Ms. Thomas has a history of multiple somatic complaints lasting at least 6 months, along with a high level of anxiety about her symptoms and excessive time and energy devoted to her health concerns. She has had multiple medical procedures and significant impairment in her social and occupational functioning.

WARDS TIP

Approximately 5–7% of the general population have a somatic symptom disorder.

Somatic Symptom Disorder

Patients with somatic symptom disorder present with at least one (and often multiple) physical symptom. They frequently seek treatment from many doctors, often resulting in extensive lab work, diagnostic procedures, hospitalizations, and/or surgeries.

DIAGNOSIS AND DSM-5 CRITERIA

- One or more somatic symptoms (may be predominantly pain) that are distressing or result in significant disruption.
- Excessive thoughts, feelings, or behaviors related to the somatic symptoms or associated health concerns.
- Lasts at least 6 months.

EPIDEMIOLOGY

- Incidence in females likely greater than that of males.
- Prevalence in general adult population: 5–7%.
- Risk factors include older age, fewer years of education, lower socioeconomic status, unemployment, and history of childhood sexual abuse.

TREATMENT AND PROGNOSIS

- The course tends to be chronic and debilitating. Symptoms may periodically improve and then worsen under stress.
- The patient should have regularly scheduled visits with a single primary care physician, who should minimize unnecessary medical workups and treatments.
- Address psychological issues slowly. Patients will likely resist referral to a mental health professional.

Conversion Disorder (Functional Neurological Symptom Disorder)

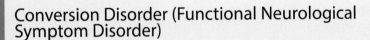

- Patients with conversion disorder have at least one neurological symptom (sensory or motor).
- Cannot be fully explained by a neurological condition.
- Patients are often surprisingly calm and unconcerned (*la belle indifference*) when describing their symptoms.
- Examples of neurological symptoms include blindness, paralysis, and paresthesia.

DIAGNOSIS AND DSM-5 CRITERIA

- At least one symptom of altered voluntary motor or sensory function.
- Evidence of incompatibility between the symptom and recognized neurological or medical conditions.
- Not better explained by another medical or mental disorder.
- Causes significant distress or impairment in social or occupational functioning or warrants medical evaluation.
- **Common symptoms:** Paralysis, weakness, blindness, mutism, sensory complaints (paresthesias), seizures, globus sensation (*globus hystericus* or sensation of lump in throat).

EPIDEMIOLOGY

- Two to three times more common in women than men
- Onset at any age, but more often in adolescence or early adulthood
- High incidence of comorbid neurological, depressive, or anxiety disorders

TREATMENT AND PROGNOSIS

- The primary treatment is education about the illness. Cognitive-behavioral therapy (CBT), with or without physical therapy, can be used if education alone is not effective.
- While patients often spontaneously recover, the prognosis is poor, as symptoms may persist, recur, or worsen in 40–66% of patients.

Illness Anxiety Disorder

DIAGNOSIS AND DSM-5 CRITERIA

- Preoccupation with having or acquiring a serious illness
- Somatic symptoms are not present or, if present, are mild in intensity
- High level of anxiety about health
- Performs excessive health-related behaviors or exhibits maladaptive behaviors
- Persists for at least **6 months**
- Not better explained by another mental disorder (such as somatic symptom disorder)

KEY FACT

Illness anxiety disorder is the only somatic symptom-related disorder that doesn't likely have a higher frequency in women.

EPIDEMIOLOGY

- Men are affected as often as women.
- Average age of onset: 20–30.
- Approximately 67% have a coexisting major mental disorder.

TREATMENT

- Regularly scheduled visits to one primary care physician.
- CBT is the most useful of psychotherapies.
- Comorbid anxiety and depressive disorders should be treated with selective serotonin reuptake inhibitors (SSRIs) or other appropriate psychotropic medications.

PROGNOSIS

- Chronic but episodic—symptoms may wax and wane periodically.
- Can result in significant disability.
- Up to 60% of patients improve significantly.
- Better prognostic factors include fewer somatic symptoms, shorter duration of illness, and absence of childhood physical punishment.

Psychological Factors Affecting Other Medical Conditions

- A patient with one or more psychological or behavioral factors (e.g., distress, coping styles, maladaptive health behaviors) adversely affecting a medical symptom or condition.
- Examples include anxiety worsening asthma, denial of need for treatment for acute chest pain, and manipulating insulin doses in order to lose weight.

DIAGNOSIS AND DSM-5 CRITERIA

- A medical symptom or condition (other than mental disorder) is present.
- Psychological or behavioral factors adversely affect the medical condition in at least one way, such as influencing the course or treatment, constituting an additional health risk factor, influencing the underlying pathophysiology, precipitating, or exacerbating symptoms or necessitating medical attention.
- Psychological or behavioral factors not better explained by another mental disorder.

EPIDEMIOLOGY

- Prevalence and gender differences are unclear.
- Can occur across the life span.

TREATMENT AND PROGNOSIS

- Treatment includes education and frequent contact with a primary care physician.
- SSRIs and/or psychotherapy (especially CBT) should be used to treat underlying anxiety or depression.

Factitious Disorder

- Patients with factitious disorder intentionally falsify medical or psychological signs or symptoms in order to assume the role of a sick patient.
- They often do this in a way that can cause legitimate danger (central line infections, insulin injections, etc.).
- The *absence of external rewards* is a prominent feature of this disorder.

DIAGNOSIS AND DSM-5 CRITERIA

- Falsification of physical or psychological signs or symptoms, or induction of injury or disease, associated with identified deception.
- The deceptive behavior is evident even in the absence of obvious external rewards (such as in malingering).
- Behavior is not better explained by another mental disorder, such as delusional disorder or another psychotic disorder.
- Individual can present him/herself, or another individual (as in factitious disorder imposed on another).
- **Commonly feigned symptoms:**
  - *Psychiatric*—hallucinations, depression
  - *Medical*—fever (by heating the thermometer), infection, hypoglycemia, abdominal pain, seizures, and hematuria

> **KEY FACT**
>
> Münchhausen syndrome is another, older name for factitious disorder with predominantly physical complaints. Münchhausen syndrome by proxy is intentionally producing symptoms in someone else who is under one's care (usually one's children).

EPIDEMIOLOGY

- May be at least 1% of hospitalized patients.
- More common in women.
- Higher incidence in hospital and health care workers (who have learned how to feign symptoms).
- Associated with personality disorders.
- Many patients have a history of illness and hospitalization, as well as childhood physical or sexual abuse.

TREATMENT AND PROGNOSIS

- Collect collateral information from medical treaters and family. Collaborate with primary care physician and treatment team to avoid unnecessary procedures.
- Patients may require confrontation in a nonthreatening manner; however, patients who are confronted may leave against medical advice and seek hospitalization elsewhere.
- Repeated and long-term hospitalizations are common.

Malingering

A 37-year-old patient claims that he has frequent episodes of "seizures," starts on medications, and joins an epilepsy support group. It becomes known that he is doing this in order to collect social security disability money. *Diagnosis?* **Malingering.** In contrast, in **factitious disorder**, patients look for some kind of unconscious emotional gain by playing the "sick role," such as sympathy from the physician. The fundamental difference between malingering and factitious disorder is in the intention of the patient; in malingering, the motivation is external, whereas in factitious disorder, the motivation is internal.

- Malingering involves the intentional reporting of physical or psychological symptoms in order to achieve personal gain.
- Common external motivations include avoiding the police, receiving room and board, obtaining narcotics, and receiving monetary compensation.
- Note that malingering is **not** considered to be a mental illness.

PRESENTATION

- Patients usually present with multiple vague complaints that do not conform to a known medical condition.
- They often have a long medical history with many hospital stays.
- They are generally uncooperative and refuse to accept a good prognosis even after extensive medical evaluation.
- Their symptoms improve once their desired objective is obtained.

EPIDEMIOLOGY

- Not uncommon in hospitalized patients
- Significantly more common in men than women

Review of Distinguishing Features

- **Somatic symptom disorders:** Patients *believe* they are ill and do not intentionally produce or feign symptoms.
- **Factitious disorder:** Patients intentionally produce symptoms of a psychological or physical illness because of a desire to assume the *sick role*, not for external rewards.
- **Malingering:** Patients intentionally produce or feign symptoms for *external rewards*.

CHAPTER 13

IMPULSE CONTROL DISORDERS

Intermittent Explosive Disorder	147	EPIDEMIOLOGY/ETIOLOGY	148
DIAGNOSIS AND DSM-5 CRITERIA	147	TREATMENT	148
EPIDEMIOLOGY/ETIOLOGY	147	Pyromania	148
TREATMENT	147	DIAGNOSIS AND DSM-5 CRITERIA	148
Kleptomania	147	EPIDEMIOLOGY/ETIOLOGY	148
DIAGNOSIS AND DSM-5 CRITERIA	147	TREATMENT	148

Impulse control disorders are characterized by problems in the self-control of emotions and behaviors. The behaviors violate the rights of others and/or conflict with societal norms. Impulse control disorders are not caused by another mental disorder, medical condition, or substance use.

Core qualities of the impulse control disorders are as follows:

1. Repetitive or compulsive engagement in behavior despite adverse consequences
2. Little control over the negative behavior
3. Anxiety or craving experienced prior to engagement in impulsive behavior
4. Relief or satisfaction during or after completion of the behavior

Mr. Baker is a 27-year-old married accountant who arrives at the outpatient psychiatry clinic complaining of difficulty in managing his anger. He has no prior psychiatric history, but reports that he has had difficulty controlling his temper since adolescence. He reports that he is easily angered by small occurrences, such as his wife's failing to make coffee or a coworker's forgetting a pen at work. He reacts quickly and in a volatile way, describing it as "going from 0 to 60 before I know it." Mr. Baker feels that he is unable to control his anger; on several occasions he has thrown objects and destroyed property in fits of rage, and has made threatening statements to his wife and coworkers in the past year. Because of these incidents, one coworker has recently threatened to pursue legal action.

Mr. Baker describes these episodes as brief, lasting only 10–15 minutes, and feels embarrassed shortly after the episode has transpired. He is concerned he may lose his job because of his behavior, and he worries about the fate of his relationships. He rarely drinks alcohol, and denies any history of illicit drug use.

What is his most likely diagnosis?

Based on Mr. Baker's history, his most likely diagnosis is intermittent explosive disorder. However, it is important to recognize that impulsivity is a common characteristic of other psychiatric diagnoses, and these must be ruled out prior to diagnosing a patient with this disorder.

What would be your recommended treatment?

Treatment for this disorder usually involves medications to treat impulsive aggression. These include selective serotonin reuptake inhibitors (SSRIs), fluoxetine being the most studied; and mood stabilizers, such as anticonvulsants and lithium. Individual psychotherapy is difficult and has limited efficacy given the nature of the disease and lack of individual control. However, cognitive-behavioral therapy (CBT) has been used in the treatment of anger management. Group therapy and/or family therapy may be useful to create behavior plans to help manage episodes.

What are associated laboratory findings?

Aside from a low mean 5-hydroxyindoleacetic acid (5-HIAA) concentration that has been found in the cerebrospinal fluid of some impulsive individuals, there may also be nonspecific electroencephalographic findings or abnormalities on neuropsychological testing.

Intermittent Explosive Disorder

DIAGNOSIS AND DSM-5 CRITERIA

- Recurrent behavioral outbursts resulting in verbal and/or physical aggression against people or property.

Either:
- Frequent verbal/physical outbursts (that do not result in physical damage to people, animals, or property) twice weekly for 3 months

Or:
- Rare (≥3×/year) outbursts resulting in physical damage to others, animals, or property
- Outbursts and aggression are grossly out of proportion to the triggering event or stressor.
- Outbursts are not premeditated and not committed to obtain a desired reward.
- Aggressive outbursts cause either marked distress or impairment in occupational/interpersonal functioning, or are associated with financial/legal consequences.
- Aggression is not better explained by another mental disorder, medical condition, or to the effects of a substance (drug or medication).

EPIDEMIOLOGY/ETIOLOGY

- More common in men than women.
- Onset usually in late childhood or adolescence teens and may be episodic or progress in severity until middle age.
- Genetic, perinatal, environmental, and neurobiological factors may play a role in etiology. Patients may have a history of child abuse, head trauma, or seizures.

> **KEY FACT**
>
> Low levels of serotonin in the CSF have been shown to be associated with impulsiveness and aggression.

TREATMENT

- Treatment involves use of SSRIs, anticonvulsants, or lithium.
- CBT has been shown to be effective and is often used in combination with medications.
- Group therapy and/or family therapy may be useful to create behavior plans to help manage episodes.

Kleptomania

DIAGNOSIS AND DSM-5 CRITERIA

- Failure to resist uncontrollable urges to steal objects that are not needed for personal use or monetary value.
- Increasing tension immediately prior to the theft.
- Pleasure or relief is experienced while stealing; however, intense guilt and depression are often reported by those with the disorder.

- Stealing not committed to express anger/vengeance and not in response to a delusion or hallucination.
- Objects stolen are typically given or thrown away, returned, or hoarded.

EPIDEMIOLOGY/ETIOLOGY

- 3× more common in women than men, though rare in the general population.
- Occurs in 4–24% of shoplifters.
- ↑ incidence of comorbid mood disorders, eating disorders (especially bulimia nervosa), anxiety disorders, substance use disorders, and personality disorders.
- Higher risk of OCD and substance use disorders in family members.
- Illness usually begins in adolescence and course is episodic.

TREATMENT

Treatment may include CBT (including systematic desensitization and aversive conditioning) and SSRIs. There is also some anecdotal evidence for naltrexone use.

Pyromania

DIAGNOSIS AND DSM-5 CRITERIA

- At least two episodes of deliberate fire setting.
- Tension or arousal experienced before the act, and pleasure, gratification, or relief experienced when setting fires or witnessing/participating in their aftermath.
- Fascination with, interest in, curiosity about, or attraction to fire and contexts.
- Purpose of fire setting is not for monetary gain, expression of anger or vengeance, to conceal criminal activity, as an expression of sociopolitical ideology, and is not in response to a hallucination, delusion, or impaired judgment (intoxication, neurocognitive disorder).
- Fire setting is not better explained by conduct disorder, a manic episode, or antisocial personality disorder.

EPIDEMIOLOGY/ETIOLOGY

- Rare disorder but much more common in men.
- Most begin to set fires in adolescence or early adulthood.
- High comorbidity with mood disorders, substance use disorders, gambling disorder, and conduct disorder.
- Episodes are episodic and wax and wane in frequency.

TREATMENT

Most don't go into treatment and will remain chronic. While there is no standard treatment, cognitive-behavior therapy, SSRIs, mood stabilizers, and antipsychotics have all been used.

KEY FACT

65% of patients with kleptomania suffer from bulimia nervosa.

KEY FACT

Pyromania is the impulse to start fires to relieve tension, typically with feelings of gratification or relief afterward.

NOTES

CHAPTER 14

EATING DISORDERS

Definition — 152

Anorexia Nervosa — 153

    DIAGNOSIS AND DSM-5 CRITERIA — 153

    PHYSICAL FINDINGS AND MEDICAL COMPLICATIONS — 153

    EPIDEMIOLOGY — 154

    ETIOLOGY — 154

    DIFFERENTIAL DIAGNOSIS — 154

    COURSE AND PROGNOSIS — 154

    TREATMENT — 154

Bulimia Nervosa — 155

    DIAGNOSIS AND DSM-5 CRITERIA — 155

    PHYSICAL FINDINGS AND MEDICAL COMPLICATIONS — 155

EPIDEMIOLOGY — 155

ETIOLOGY — 155

COURSE AND PROGNOSIS — 155

TREATMENT — 156

Binge-Eating Disorder — 156

    DIAGNOSIS AND DSM-5 CRITERIA — 156

    PHYSICAL FINDINGS AND MEDICAL COMPLICATIONS — 156

    EPIDEMIOLOGY — 156

    ETIOLOGY — 156

    COURSE AND PROGNOSIS — 157

    TREATMENT — 157

Definition

Eating disorders include anorexia nervosa, bulimia nervosa, and binge-eating disorder. Patients with anorexia or bulimia have a disturbed body image and use extensive measures to avoid gaining weight (vomiting, laxatives, diuretics, enemas, fasting, and excessive exercise). Patients with binge-eating disorder typically binge in response to negative emotions.

Ms. Williams is a 17-year-old Caucasian woman without prior psychiatric history who is brought to the emergency room by ambulance after her parents called 911 when they found her having a seizure in their living room. She was admitted to the medical intensive care unit in status epilepticus and was quickly stabilized with intramuscular lorazepam and fosphenytoin loading. Her height is 5 feet 6 inches, she is of medium build, and her weight is 101 pounds (BMI 16.3 kg/m^2). She has no significant medical history, and this is her first seizure. Laboratory workup shows an electrolyte imbalance as the most likely cause for her seizures. Although initially reluctant, she admits to purging with the use of ipecac several times this week. She reports that although she normally restricts her daily caloric intake to 500 calories, she regularly induces vomiting if her weight is above 100 pounds. Her last menstrual cycle was 1 year ago. Psychiatric consultation is requested in order to confirm her diagnosis.

As the psychiatrist on call, you evaluate Ms. Williams and find that she appears underweight and younger than her stated age. She is in mild distress, has a nasogastric tube in place, and exhibits poor eye contact. She reports feeling "sad" and admits to experiencing constant preoccupation about her physical appearance, stating "I'm fat; I hate my body." She also reports insomnia, low energy levels, and a history of self-harm behavior by cutting her forearms. She reports that she is careful in hiding her symptoms from her parents, whom she describes as strict disciplinarians. She also expresses concerns that she will disappoint them.

Ms. Williams's parents describe her as a perfectionist. They say that she is involved in multiple school activities, takes advanced placement classes, and has been recently concerned about being accepted to her college of choice. They report that she has maintained a 4.0 grade point average in high school, and they expect her to become a doctor. Her parents have noticed that she is underweight and rarely see her eat, but have attributed this to stress from her many academic pursuits. Ms. Williams's mother receives treatment for obsessive-compulsive disorder.

What is Ms. Williams's most likely diagnosis?

The most likely diagnosis is anorexia nervosa—binge-eating/purging type. As described above, she refuses to weigh more than 100 pounds, which is significantly below the minimal normal weight for her height. Despite being underweight, she expresses intense fear of gaining weight and has a disturbance in the way her body shape is experienced. In addition, she has engaged in binge-eating/purging behavior regularly. You should also explore for comorbid depression, anxiety, and a personality disorder. Remember that malnutrition in itself can lead to some of the symptoms experienced in depression, and that many patients show an improvement in their mood when nutrition is replenished.

What are some of the medical complications associated with this condition?

Patients with anorexia nervosa might present with bradycardia, orthostatic hypotension, arrhythmias, QTc prolongation, and ST-T wave changes on electrocardiogram, as well as anemia and leukopenia. They might also experience cognitive impairment, evidence of enlarged ventricles and/or ↓ gray and white matter on brain imaging, and peripheral neuropathy. Lanugo and muscle wasting sometimes become evident. Amenorrhea and loss of libido are commonly reported. In patients who regularly engage in self-induced vomiting, parotid enlargement, ↑ amylase levels, and electrolyte imbalances (e.g., hypokalemia) commonly occur as a result.

Anorexia Nervosa

Patients with anorexia nervosa are preoccupied with their weight, their body image, and being thin. It is often associated with obsessive-compulsive personality traits. There are two main sub types:

- **Restricting type:** Has not regularly engaged in binge-eating or purging behavior; weight loss is achieved through diet, fasting, and/or excessive exercise.
- **Binge-eating/purging type:** Eating binges followed by self-induced vomiting, and/or using laxatives, enemas, or diuretics. Some individuals purge after eating small amounts of food without binging.

DIAGNOSIS AND DSM-5 CRITERIA

- Restriction of energy intake relative to requirements, leading to significant low body weight—defined as less than minimally normal or expected
- Intense fear of gaining weight or becoming fat, or persistent behaviors that prevent weight gain
- Disturbed body image, undue influence of weight or shape on self-evaluation, or denial of the seriousness of the current low body weight

PHYSICAL FINDINGS AND MEDICAL COMPLICATIONS

- The medical complications of eating disorders are related to weight loss and purging (e.g., vomiting and laxative abuse).
- Physical manifestations: Amenorrhea, cold intolerance/hypothermia, hypotension (especially orthostasis), bradycardia, arrhythmia, acute coronary syndrome, cardiomyopathy, mitral valve prolapse, constipation, lanugo hair, alopecia, edema, dehydration, peripheral neuropathy, seizures, hypothyroidism, osteopenia, osteoporosis.
- Laboratory/imaging abnormalities: Hyponatremia, hypochloremic hypokalemic alkalosis (if vomiting), arrhythmia (especially QTc prolongation), hypercholesterolemia, transaminitis, leukopenia, anemia (normocytic normochromic), elevated blood urea nitrogen (BUN), ↑ growth hormone (GH), ↑ cortisol, reduced gonadotropins (luteinizing hormone [LH], follicle-stimulating hormone [FSH]), reduced sex steroid hormones (estrogen, testosterone), hypothyroidism, hypoglycemia, osteopenia.

KEY FACT

Both anorexia and bulimia are characterized by a desire for thinness. Both may binge and purge. Anorexia nervosa involves low body weight and restriction of calorie intake, and this distinguishes it from bulimia.

KEY FACT

Classic example of anorexia nervosa: An extremely thin amenorrheic teenage girl whose mother says she eats very little, does aerobics for 2 hours a day, and *ritualistically* performs 400 sit-ups every day (500 if she has "overeaten").

EPIDEMIOLOGY

- 10 to 1 female to male ratio. Twelve-month prevalence among young females is 0.4%.
- Bimodal age of onset (age 13–14: hormonal influences; age 17–18: environmental influences). More common in industrialized countries where food is abundant and a thin body ideal is held.
- Common in sports that involve thinness, revealing attire, subjective judging, and weight classes (e.g., running, ballet, wrestling, diving, cheerleading, figure skating).

ETIOLOGY

- Multifactorial.
- Genetics: Higher concordance in monozygotic than dizygotic twin studies.
- Psychodynamic theories: Difficulty with separation and autonomy (e.g., parental enmeshment), and struggle to gain control.
- Social theories: Exaggeration of social values (achievement, control, and perfectionism), idealization of thin body and prepubescent appearance in Western world, ↑ prevalence of dieting at earlier ages.

DIFFERENTIAL DIAGNOSIS

- Medical conditions: Endocrine disorders (e.g., hypothalamic disease, diabetes mellitus, hyperthyroidism), gastrointestinal illnesses (e.g., malabsorption, inflammatory bowel disease), genetic disorders (e.g., Turner syndrome, Gaucher disease), cancer, AIDS.
- Psychiatric disorders: Major depression, bulimia, or other mental disorders (such as somatic symptom disorder or schizophrenia).

COURSE AND PROGNOSIS

- Chronic and relapsing illness. Variable course—may completely recover, have fluctuating symptoms with relapses, or progressively deteriorate. Most remit within 5 years.
- Mortality rate is cumulative and approximately 5% per decade due to starvation, **suicide**, or cardiac failure. Rates of suicide are approximately 12 per 100,000 per year.

TREATMENT

- Food is the best medicine!
- Patients may be treated as outpatients unless they are dangerously below ideal body weight (>20–25% below) or if there are serious medical or psychiatric complications, in which case they should be hospitalized for supervised refeeding.
- Treatment involves cognitive-behavioral therapy, family therapy (e.g., Maudsley approach), and supervised weight-gain programs.
- Selective serotonin reuptake inhibitors (SSRIs) have not been effective in the treatment of anorexia nervosa but may be used for comorbid anxiety or depression.
- Little evidence that second-generation antipsychotics can treat preoccupation with weight and food, or independently promote weight gain.

KEY FACT

Anorexia versus Major Depressive Disorder: Appetite
Anorexia nervosa: Patients have a *good appetite* but starve themselves due to distorted body image. They are often quite preoccupied with food (e.g., preparing it for others) but do not eat it themselves.
Major depressive disorder: Patients usually have *poor appetite*, which leads to weight loss. These patients have no or decreased interest in food.

KEY FACT

Refeeding syndrome refers to electrolyte and fluid shifts that occur when severely malnourished patients are refed too quickly. Look for fluid retention and ↓ levels of phosphorus, magnesium, and calcium. Complications include arrhythmias, respiratory failure, delirium, and seizures. Replace electrolytes and slow the feedings.

WARDS TIP

When a patient with anorexia learns that weight gain is a common side effect, he/she may refuse medication.

Bulimia Nervosa

Bulimia nervosa involves binge eating combined with behaviors intended to counteract weight gain, such as vomiting; use of laxatives, enemas, or diuretics; fasting; or excessive exercise. Patients are embarrassed by their binge eating and are overly concerned with body weight. However, unlike patients with anorexia, they usually maintain a normal weight (and may be overweight).

DIAGNOSIS AND DSM-5 CRITERIA

- Recurrent episodes of binge eating.
- Recurrent, inappropriate attempts to compensate for overeating and prevent weight gain (such as laxative abuse, vomiting, diuretics, fasting, or excessive exercise).
- The binge eating and compensatory behaviors occur at least once a week for 3 months.
- Perception of self-worth is excessively influenced by body weight and shape.
- Does not occur exclusively during an episode of anorexia nervosa.

PHYSICAL FINDINGS AND MEDICAL COMPLICATIONS

- Patients with anorexia and bulimia may have similar medical complications related to weight loss and vomiting.
- Physical manifestations: Salivary gland enlargement (sialadenosis), dental erosion/caries, callouses/abrasions on dorsum of hand ("Russell's sign" from self-induced vomiting), petechiae, peripheral edema, aspiration.
- Laboratory/imaging abnormalities: Hypochloremic hypokalemic alkalosis, metabolic acidosis (laxative abuse), elevated bicarbonate (compensation), hypernatremia, ↑ BUN, ↑ amylase, altered thyroid hormone, cortisol homeostasis, and esophagitis.

EPIDEMIOLOGY

- 12-month prevalence in young females is 1–1.5%.
- Significantly more common in women than men (10:1 ratio).
- Onset is in late adolescence or early adulthood.
- More common in developed countries.
- High incidence of comorbid mood disorders, anxiety disorders, impulse control disorders, substance use, prior physical/sexual abuse, and ↑ prevalence of borderline personality disorder.

ETIOLOGY

- Multifactorial, with similar factors as for anorexia (e.g., genetic and social theories)
- Childhood obesity and early pubertal maturation increase risk for bulimia nervosa
- Psychodynamic theories: Masochistic displays of control and displaced anger over one's body

COURSE AND PROGNOSIS

- Chronic and relapsing illness.
- Better prognosis than anorexia nervosa.

WARDS TIP

Unlike patients with anorexia nervosa, bulimic patients usually maintain a normal weight (or are overweight) and their symptoms are more ego-dystonic (distressing); they are therefore more likely to seek help.

KEY FACT

Binge eating is defined by excessive food intake within a 2-hour period accompanied by a sense of lack of control.

KEY FACT

Cortisol is often ↑ in patients with anorexia nervosa.

KEY FACT

Anorexia nervosa and bulimia nervosa are risk factors for developing cardiac arrhythmias due to electrolyte disturbances such as hypokalemia.

- Symptoms are usually exacerbated by stressful conditions.
- One-half recover fully with treatment; one-half have chronic course with fluctuating symptoms.
- Crude mortality rate is 2% per decade.
- Elevated suicide risk compared to the general population.

TREATMENT

- Antidepressants plus therapy (more effective combo for bulimia than for anorexia).
- SSRIs are first-line medication.
- Fluoxetine is the only FDA-approved medication for bulimia (60–80 mg/day).
- Nutritional counseling and education.
- Therapy includes cognitive-behavioral therapy, interpersonal psychotherapy, group therapy, and family therapy.
- Avoid bupropion due to its potential side effect to lower seizure threshold.

Binge-Eating Disorder

Patients with binge-eating disorder suffer emotional distress over their binge eating, but they do not try to control their weight by purging or restricting calories, as do anorexics or bulimics. Unlike anorexia and bulimia, patients with binge-eating disorder are not as fixated on their body shape and weight.

DIAGNOSIS AND DSM-5 CRITERIA

- Recurrent episodes of binge eating (eating an excessive amount of food in a 2-hour period associated with a lack of control), with at least three of the following: eating very rapidly, eating until uncomfortably full, eating large amounts when not hungry, eating alone due to embarrassment, and feeling disgusted/depressed/guilty after eating.
- Severe distress over binge eating.
- Binge eating occurs at least once a week for 3 months.
- Binge eating is not associated with compensatory behaviors (such as vomiting, laxative use, etc.), and doesn't occur exclusively during the course of anorexia or bulimia.

PHYSICAL FINDINGS AND MEDICAL COMPLICATIONS

Patients are typically obese and suffer from medical problems related to obesity including metabolic syndrome, type II diabetes, and cardiovascular disease.

EPIDEMIOLOGY

- Twelve-month prevalence is 1.6% for females and 0.8% for males
- Equal prevalence in females across ethnicities
- Increased prevalence among individuals seeking weight-loss treatment compared to the general population

ETIOLOGY

Runs in families, reflecting likely genetic influences

COURSE AND PROGNOSIS

- Typically begins in adolescence or young adulthood
- Appears to be relatively persistent though remission rates are higher than for other eating disorders
- Most obese individuals do not binge eat; those who do have more functional impairment, lower quality of life, and more subjective distress than weight matched controls
- Higher rates of psychiatric comorbidities than in obese individuals without binge eating disorder

TREATMENT

- Treatment involves individual (cognitive-behavioral or interpersonal) psychotherapy with a strict diet and exercise program. Comorbid mood disorders or anxiety disorders should be treated as necessary.
- Although their utility is limited by significant side effects and limited evidence, pharmacotherapy may be used adjunctively to promote weight loss:
  - Stimulants (such as phentermine and amphetamine)—suppress appetite.
  - Topiramate and zonisimide—antiepileptics associated with weight loss.
  - Orlistat (Xenical)—inhibits pancreatic lipase, thus decreasing amount of fat absorbed from gastrointestinal tract.

NOTES

CHAPTER 15

SLEEP-WAKE DISORDERS

Normal Sleep-Wake Cycle   160

Sleep Disorders   160

Dyssomnias   160

    Insomnia Disorder   160

    Hypersomnolence Disorder   161

    Obstructive Sleep Apnea Hypopnea   162

    Central Sleep Apnea   163

    Sleep-Related Hypoventilation   163

    Narcolepsy   165

    Circadian Rhythm Sleep-Wake Disorders   165

Parasomnias   166

    Non-REM Sleep Arousal Disorders   166

    Sleepwalking   167

    Sleep Terrors   167

    Nightmare Disorder   168

    REM Sleep Behavior Disorder   168

    Restless Legs Syndrome   169

Sleep disorders affect as many as 40% of the US adult population. Current data demonstrate a high rate of comorbidity between sleep disorders and various psychiatric illnesses. Disturbances in sleep can potentiate and/or exacerbate psychological distress and other mental illnesses.

Normal Sleep-Wake Cycle

- Normal sleep-wake cycle is defined in terms of characteristic changes in several physiological parameters, including brain wave activity, eye movements, and motor activity.
- The two stages of normal sleep are rapid eye movement (REM) sleep and non–rapid eye movement (NREM) sleep.
- About every 90 minutes, NREM sleep alternates with REM sleep.
- NREM induces transition from the waking state to deep sleep.
- Progression through NREM sleep results in slower brain wave patterns and higher arousal thresholds.
- In REM sleep, brain wave patterns resemble the electroencephalogram (EEG) of an aroused person.
- Awakening from REM sleep is associated with vivid dream recall.

Sleep Disorders

- Classified as either:
  - **Dyssomnias:** Insufficient, excessive, or altered timing of sleep
  - **Parasomnias:** Unusual sleep-related behaviors
- When taking a sleep history, ask about:
  - **A**ctivities prior to bedtime that may interfere with restful sleep
  - **B**ed partner history
  - **C**onsequence on waking function; quality of life
  - **D**rug regimen, medications
  - **E**xacerbating or relieving factors
  - **F**requency and duration
  - **G**enetic factors or family history
  - **H**abits (alcohol consumption, use of caffeine, nicotine, illicit substances, and hypnotics)

Dyssomnias

Dyssomnias are disorders that make it difficult to fall or remain asleep (insomnias), or of excessive daytime sleeping (hypersomnias).

INSOMNIA DISORDER

- Refers to number of symptoms that interfere with duration and/or quality of sleep despite adequate opportunity for sleep. Symptoms may include:
  - Difficulty initiating sleep (*initial or sleep-onset insomnia*)
  - Frequent nocturnal awakenings (*middle or sleep-maintenance insomnia*)
  - Early morning awakenings (*late or sleep-offset insomnia*)
  - Waking up feeling fatigued and unrefreshed (*nonrestorative sleep*)
- **Acute insomnia** (less than 3 months) is generally associated with stress or changes in sleep schedule and usually resolves spontaneously.
- **Chronic insomnia** lasts ≥3 months to years and is associated with reduced quality of life and ↑ risk of psychiatric illness.

WARDS TIP

Breathing-related disorders are the most common of the hypersomnias and include obstructive sleep apnea and central sleep apnea.

DSM-5 Criteria

- Difficulty initiating/maintaining sleep or early-morning awakening with inability to return to sleep
- Occurs at least 3 days a week for at least 3 months
- Causes clinically significant distress or impairment in functioning
- Occurs despite adequate opportunity to sleep
- Does not occur exclusively during the course of another sleep-wake disorder
- Not due to the physiologic effects of a substance or medication
- Coexisting mental and medical disorders do not adequately explain the insomnia

Epidemiology

Prevalence: 6–10% (the most prevalent of all sleep-wake disorders).

Etiology

- Subclinical mood and/or anxiety disorders
- Preoccupation with a perceived inability to sleep
- Bedtime behavior not conducive to adequate sleep (**poor sleep hygiene**)
- Idiopathic

Treatment

- Sleep hygiene measures
- Cognitive-behavioral therapy (CBT)
- Pharmacotherapy:
  - Benzodiazepines:
    - Reduce sleep latency and nocturnal awakening.
    - As effective as CBT during short periods of treatment (4–8 weeks); insufficient evidence to support long-term efficacy.
    - Side effects include development of tolerance, addiction, daytime sleepiness, and rebound insomnia.
    - In the elderly, falls, confusion, and dizziness are of particular concern.
  - Non-benzodiazepines:
    - Include zolpidem (Ambien), eszopiclone (Lunesta), and zaleplon (Sonata).
    - Effective for short-term treatment.
    - Associated with low incidence of daytime sleepiness and orthostatic hypotension.
    - In the elderly, zolpidem causes ↑ risk of falls and may induce cognitive impairment.
    - Doses of zolpidem >10 mg can cause ↑ cognitive impairment in women.
  - Antidepressants:
    - Trazodone, amitriptyline, and doxepin (off-label use).
    - Side effects include sedation, dizziness, and psychomotor impairment.
    - Trazodone is the most prescribed sedating antidepressant for patients with chronic insomnia and depressive symptoms.

> **KEY FACT**
>
> CBT is considered first-line therapy for chronic insomnia.

> **KEY FACT**
>
> Insomnia is the most common reason patients are put on long-term benzodiazepines.

> **KEY FACT**
>
> REM sleep is characterized by ↑ in blood pressure, heart rate, and respiratory rate.

HYPERSOMNOLENCE DISORDER

- Refers to symptoms of excessive quantity of sleep, reduced quality of wakefulness, and sleep inertia/*sleep drunkenness* (i.e., impaired performance and reduced alertness after awakening).
- Complain of nonrestorative sleep, automatic behaviors (routine behavior performed with little to no recall), and difficulty awakening in the morning.

DSM-5 Criteria

- Excessive sleepiness despite at least 7 hours of sleep, with at least one of the following: recurrent periods of sleep within the same day; prolonged, nonrestorative sleep >9 hours; difficulty being fully awake after awakening
- Occurs at least 3 times per week for at least 3 months
- Causes clinically significant distress or impairment in functioning
- Does not occur exclusively during the course of another sleep-wake disorder
- Not due to the physiologic effects of a substance or medication
- Coexisting mental and medical disorders do not adequately explain the hypersomnolence

Epidemiology

Prevalence: 5–10% of individuals presenting to sleep disorders clinics.
Equal frequency in men and women.

Etiology

- Viral infections (e.g., HIV pneumonia, infectious mononucleosis, Guillain–Barré)
- Head trauma
- Genetic—may have autosomal dominant mode of inheritance in some individuals

Course

- Progressive onset, beginning between ages 15 and 25
- Persistent course unless treated

Treatment

- Life-long therapy with modafinil or stimulants such as methylphenidate; amphetamine-like antidepressants such as atomoxetine are second-line therapy
- Scheduled napping

OBSTRUCTIVE SLEEP APNEA HYPOPNEA

A 40-year-old businessman states that over the past 2 years he has had trouble staying awake for more than 2 hours before eventually falling asleep. He then has a hard time sleeping through the night. As a result, his performance at work is suffering. *Diagnosis?* Many possible diagnoses, but you must always consider obstructive sleep apnea in addition to insomnia disorder, narcolepsy, etc.

Chronic breathing-related disorder characterized by repetitive collapse of the upper airway during sleep and evidence by polysomnography of multiple episodes of apnea or hypopnea per hour of sleep.

Features

- Excessive daytime sleepiness
- Apneic episodes characterized by cessation of breathing or hypopneic episodes of reduced airflow (>15 per hour)

- Sleep fragmentation
- Snoring
- Frequent awakenings due to gasping or choking
- Nonrefreshing sleep or fatigue
- Morning headaches
- Hypertension

Risk Factors

Obesity, ↑ neck circumference, airway narrowing.

Prevalence

- Most common in middle-aged men and women
- Male to female ratio ranges from 2:1 to 4:1
- Children: 1–2%; middle-aged adults: 2–15%; older adults: >20%

Treatment

- Positive airway pressure: continuous (CPAP) and in some cases bilevel (BiPAP)
- Behavioral strategies such as weight loss and exercise
- Surgery

CENTRAL SLEEP APNEA

Evidenced by five or more central apneas per hour of sleep. It can be idiopathic, with Cheyne–Stokes breathing (pattern of periodic crescendo–decrescendo variation in tidal volume due to heart failure, stroke, or renal failure), or due to opioid use. It is associated with insomnia and daytime sleepiness.

Prevalence

- Idiopathic subtype rare.
- Cheyne–Stokes subtype high in patients with decreased ejection fraction and acute stroke.
- 30% of chronic opioid users have central sleep apnea.
- Higher frequency in men than women.

Course

- Tied to comorbid medical conditions, although may be transient
- May be chronic in opioid users

Treatment

- Treat the underlying condition
- CPAP/BiPAP
- Supplemental O_2
- Medications (e.g., Acetazolamide [Diamox], Theophylline, sedative-hypnotics)

SLEEP-RELATED HYPOVENTILATION

Polysomnography demonstrates decreased respiration and elevated CO_2 levels. Individuals report frequent arousals, morning headaches, insomnia, and excessive daytime sleepiness. Frequently comorbid with medical or neurologic disorders, medication use, or substance use disorder. Over time it can result in pulmonary hypertension, cor pulmonale, cardiac arrhythmias, polycythemia, neurocognitive dysfunction, and eventually respiratory failure due to severe blood gas abnormalities.

Prevalence

Very uncommon

Course

Slowly progressive

Treatment

- Treat the underlying condition
- CPAP/BiPAP
- Medications to stimulate/promote breathing (e.g., bronchodilators, Theophylline)

Mr. Richards is a 22-year-old college student with a history of persistent depressive disorder (dysthymic disorder) who arrives at the outpatient psychiatry clinic complaining of daytime sleepiness. He reports that during the past 2 years, he has fallen asleep while in social situations and during his college classes. He often takes naps during class, in movie theaters, and sometimes in the middle of conversations with his girlfriend. His naps typically last for 5–10 minutes and he awakens feeling better. However, within the next 2–3 hours he feels sleepy again. His colleagues joke about his tendency to sleep everywhere, and he feels embarrassed by this.

Mr. Richards also complains of "weird" experiences while sleeping. He reports that he sometimes sees bright colors and hears loud sounds that feel real to him. He says that when this occurs it is difficult to distinguish if he is dreaming or is awake. He feels frightened by these experiences because he is unable to move when they happen. However, after a few minutes he reports that these feelings resolve, and he is able to move and is fully awake.

In performing a thorough history, you learn that he has had episodes during which he has experienced weakness and has dropped objects from his hands while laughing or becoming angry. Last week, his legs buckled and he fell to the ground after his friends surprised him at a surprise birthday party. He denies ever losing consciousness during these episodes, and there have been no reports of witnessed convulsions.

What is this patient's diagnosis?

This patient's symptoms are consistent with a diagnosis of narcolepsy. The classic narcolepsy tetrad (all four present in <25% of patients) consists of excessive daytime sleepiness or "sleep attacks," REM-related sleep phenomena including inability to move during the transition from sleep to wakefulness, hypnagogic or hypnopompic hallucinations, and a sudden loss of muscle tone evoked by strong emotion without loss of consciousness (cataplexy). Cataplexy may be mild, affecting only the voice, face, or arms, or generalized, causing patients to fall to the ground, and it occurs in 70% of those diagnosed with narcolepsy.

What are Mr. Richards's treatment options?

In the treatment of narcolepsy, it is important for patients to schedule daytime naps and to maintain a regular sleep schedule at night. They should get at least 8 hours of sleep and keep consistent times for sleeping and awakening. Pharmacological treatments may include the use of stimulants (methylphenidate) and antidepressants. The stimulant modafinil and sodium oxybate (non-stimulant) are also effective in the treatment of narcolepsy. Sodium oxybate (Xyrem) is particularly effective in the treatment of cataplexy.

NARCOLEPSY

Narcolepsy is characterized by excessive daytime sleepiness and falling asleep at inappropriate times.

DSM-5 criteria

- Recurrent episodes of need to sleep, lapsing into sleep, or napping during the day, occurring at least 3 times per week for at least 3 months associated with at least one of the following:
    - Cataplexy (brief episodes of sudden bilateral loss of muscle tone, most often associated with intense emotion)
    - Hypocretin deficiency in the CSF
    - Reduced REM sleep latency on polysomnography
- Hallucinations and/or sleep paralysis at the beginning or end of sleep episodes are common (but not necessary for diagnosis in the *DSM-5*)

Epidemiology/Prevalence

- Narcolepsy with cataplexy occurs in 0.02–0.04% worldwide.
- Slightly more common in males than females.

Pathophysiology

- Linked to a loss of hypothalamic neurons that produce hypocretin
- May have autoimmune component

Treatment

- Sleep hygiene
- Scheduled daytime naps
- Avoidance of shift work
- For excessive daytime sleepiness:
    - Amphetamines (D-amphetamine, methamphetamine)
    - Non-amphetamines such as methylphenidate, modafinil, and sodium oxybate
- For cataplexy:
    - Sodium oxybate (drug of choice)
    - Tricyclic antidepressants (TCAs): Imipramine, desipramine, and clomipramine
    - Selective serotonin reuptake inhibitor (SSRI)/serotonin-norepinephrine reuptake inhibitor (SNRI): Fluoxetine, duloxetine, atomoxetine, venlafaxine

CIRCADIAN RHYTHM SLEEP-WAKE DISORDERS

Circadian rhythm sleep wake disorders are recurrent patterns of sleep disruption due to an alteration of the circadian system or misalignment between the endogenous circadian rhythm and sleep-wake schedule required by an individual's environment or schedule. Subtypes include delayed sleep phase,

KEY FACT

Hypnagogic hallucination: when *going to* sleep.

KEY FACT

Hyponopomic hallucination: when transitioning *from* sleep.

KEY FACT

Don't confuse narcoleptic cataplexy with catatonic catalepsy (unprovoked muscular rigidity).

TABLE 15-1. Circadian Rhythm Sleep Wake Disorders

DISORDER	DEFINITION	RISK FACTORS	TREATMENTS
Delayed sleep phase disorder (DPSD)	Chronic or recurrent delay in sleep onset and awakening times with preserved quality and duration of sleep	■ Puberty (secondary to temporal changes in melatonin secretion) ■ Caffeine and nicotine use ■ Irregular sleep schedules	■ Timed bright light phototherapy during early morning ■ Administration of melatonin in the evening ■ Chronotherapy (delaying bedtime by a few hours each night)
Advanced sleep phase disorder	Normal duration and quality of sleep with sleep onset and awakening times earlier than desired	Older age	■ Timed bright light phototherapy prior to bedtime ■ Early morning melatonin not recommended (may cause daytime sedation)
Shift-work disorder (SWD)	Sleep deprivation and misalignment of the circadian rhythm secondary to nontraditional work hours	■ Night shift work ■ Rotating shifts ■ Shifts >16 hours ■ *Being a medical/psychiatry resident*	■ Avoid risk factors ■ Bright light phototherapy to facilitate rapid adaptation to night shift ■ Modafinil may be helpful for patients with severe SWD
Jet lag disorder	Sleep disturbances (insomnia, hypersomnia) associated with travel across multiple time zones	Recent sleep deprivation	■ Disorder is usually self-limiting. ■ Sleep disturbances generally resolve 2–3 days after travel.

advanced sleep phase, irregular sleep-wake, non-24-hour sleep-wake, and shift work (see Table 15-1).

Symptoms

- Excessive daytime sleepiness
- Insomnia
- Sleep inertia
- Headaches
- Difficulty concentrating
- ↑ reaction times and frequent performance errors
- Irritability
- Waking up at inappropriate times

Parasomnias

- Abnormal behaviors, experiences, or physiological events that occur during sleep or sleep-wake transitions.
- Symptoms may include abnormal movements, emotions, dreams, and autonomic activity.
- Isolated episodes common in childhood and adolescence.

NON-REM SLEEP AROUSAL DISORDERS

Repeated episodes of incomplete arousals that are brief and usually occur during the first third of the sleep episode. Include sleepwalking and sleep terrors.

SLEEPWALKING

Features

- Repeated episodes of simple to complex behaviors that occur during slow-wave sleep.
- Behaviors may include sitting up in bed, walking around, eating, and in some cases "escaping" outdoors.
- Eyes are usually open with a blank stare and "glassy look."
- Difficulty arousing the sleepwalker during an episode.
- Dreams aren't remembered and there is amnesia for the episode.
- Episodes usually end with patients returning to bed or awakening (briefly) confused and disoriented.
- Rare cases associated with violent behavior.

Epidemiology

- 1–7% of adults have sleepwalking episodes (not disorder)
- 10–30% of children have at least one episode and 2–3% sleepwalk often

Risk Factors

- Sleep deprivation
- Irregular sleep schedules
- Stress
- Fatigue
- Obstructive sleep apnea
- Nocturnal seizures
- Fever
- Medications, including sedatives/hypnotics, lithium, and anticholinergics
- Family history

Etiology

- Unknown
- Family history in 80% of cases
- Usually not associated with any significant underlying psychiatric or psychological problems

Treatment

- Most cases do not need to be treated.
- Patients may benefit from education, reassurance, addressing precipitating factors, ensuring a safe environment, and proper sleep hygiene.
- Refractory cases may respond to low-dose benzodiazepine (e.g., clonazepam).

SLEEP TERRORS

Features

- Recurrent episodes of sudden terror arousals, usually beginning with screaming or crying, that occur during slow-wave sleep.
- Signs of autonomic arousal, including tachycardia, tachypnea, diaphoresis, and mydriasis.
- Difficulty arousing during an episode.
- After episode, patients usually return to sleep without awakening.
- Dreams aren't remembered and there is amnesia for the episode.
- In rare cases, awakening elicits aggressive behavior.

Epidemiology

- Approximately 2% of adults and 20% of young children have sleep terrors (not disorder).
- 10-fold increase in first-degree biological relatives of affected patients.
- High comorbidity with sleepwalking.

Risk Factors

- Same as for sleepwalking
- Other sleep disorder such as sleep apnea

Treatment

- Reassurance that the condition is benign and self-limited.
- Same as for sleepwalking.

NIGHTMARE DISORDER

Features

- Recurrent frightening dreams that occur during the second half of the sleep episode
- Terminate in awakening with vivid recall
- No confusion or disorientation upon awakening
- Causes clinically significant distress or impairment in functioning

Epidemiology

- Frequent nightmares in 1–2% of adults, higher prevalence in women.
- Peak prevalence in late adolescence or early adulthood.
- Nightmares are seen in at least 50–70% of posttraumatic stress disorder (PTSD) cases.

Treatment

- Not always needed. Reassurance may help in many cases.
- **Desensitization/Imagery rehearsal therapy** (IRT) involves the use of mental imagery to modify the outcome of a recurrent nightmare, writing down the improved outcome, and then mentally rehearsing it in a relaxed state.
- **Medications rarely indicated**, although Prazosin and antidepressants are often used to treat nightmares in PTSD.

REM SLEEP BEHAVIOR DISORDER

Features

- Repeated arousals during sleep associated with vocalization or complex motor behavior (dream enacting behaviors) occurring during REM, more often in the second half of the sleep episode
- Characterized by lack of muscle atonia during REM sleep
- No confusion or disorientation upon awakening
- Dream-enacting behaviors include:
  - Sleep talking
  - Yelling
  - Limb jerking
  - Walking and/or running
  - Punching and/or other violent behaviors
- Presenting complaint is often violent behaviors during sleep resulting in injury to the patient and/or to the bed partner.

WARDS TIP

Imagery rehearsal therapy (IRT) has been successful in treating recurrent nightmares in patients with PTSD.

Epidemiology

- Prevalence in general population is approximately 0.5%, likely higher in people with psychiatric disorders
- Occurs mostly in males

Risk Factors

- Older age, generally > 50
- Psychiatric medications such as TCAs, SSRIs, SNRIs, and β-blockers
- Narcolepsy
- Highly associated with underlying neurodegenerative disorders, especially Parkinson's, multiple system atrophy, and neurocognitive disorder with Lewy bodies

Treatment

- Discontinuation of likely causative medications if possible.
- Clonazepam is efficacious in most patients.
- Melatonin may also be helpful.
- Ensure environmental safety such as removing potentially dangerous objects from the bedroom and sleeping on the ground until behaviors can be managed effectively.

RESTLESS LEGS SYNDROME

Features

- The urge to move legs accompanied by unpleasant sensation in the legs, characterized by relief with movement, aggravation with inactivity, and only occurring or worsening in the evening.

Epidemiology

- Prevalence is 2–7% in the general population
- Females 1.5–2× more likely than males
- Prevalence may be lower in Asian population

Risk Factors

- Increases with age
- Strong familial component
- Iron deficiency
- Antidepressants, antipsychotics, dopamine-blocking antiemetics, and anti-histamines can contribute to or worsen symptoms
- Multiple medical comorbidities, including cardiovascular disease

Treatment

- Responds well to pharmacologic treatments.
- Remove offending agents if possible.
- Iron replacement if low ferritin.
- Dopamine agonists and benzodiazepines are first-line treatments.
- Low-potency opioids can be used for treatment-refractory patients.

CHAPTER 16

SEXUAL DYSFUNCTIONS AND PARAPHILIC DISORDERS

Sexual Response Cycle   172

Sexual Changes with Aging   172

Differential Diagnosis of Sexual Dysfunctions   172

Sexual Dysfunctions   173

Treatment of Sexual Disorders   174

    SEX THERAPY   174

    COGNITIVE-BEHAVIORAL THERAPY   175

    HYPNOSIS   175

    GROUP THERAPY   175

ANALYTICALLY ORIENTED (PSYCHODYNAMIC) PSYCHOTHERAPY   175

PHARMACOLOGIC TREATMENT   175

MECHANICAL THERAPIES   175

Gender Dysphoria   176

    DIAGNOSIS AND DSM-5 CRITERIA   176

    TREATMENT   176

Paraphilias   176

    EXAMPLES OF PARAPHILIC DISORDERS   177

Sexual dysfunctions include clinically significant disturbances in individuals' ability to respond sexually or to experience sexual pleasure.

Sexual Response Cycle

There are several stages of normal sexual response in men and women:

1. **Desire:** The motivation or interest in sexual activity, often reflected by sexual fantasies.
2. **Excitement/Arousal:** Begins with either fantasy or physical contact. It is characterized by erections and testicular enlargement in men and by vaginal lubrication, clitoral erection, labial swelling, and elevation of the uterus in the pelvis (*tenting*) in women. Both men and women experience flushing, nipple erection, and increased respiration, pulse, and blood pressure.
3. **Orgasm:** In men just prior there is tightening of the scrotal sac and secretion of a few drops of seminal fluid. Women experience contraction of the outer one-third of the vagina and enlargement of the upper one-third of the vagina.

   Men ejaculate and women have contractions of the uterus and lower one-third of the vagina. There is facial grimacing, release of tension, slight clouding of consciousness, involuntary anal sphincter contractions, and acute increase in blood pressure and pulse in both men and women.
4. **Resolution:** Muscles relax and cardiovascular state returns to baseline. Detumescence of genitalia in both sexes. Men have a *refractory period* lasting minutes to hours during which they cannot reexperience orgasm; women have little or no refractory period.

Sexual Changes with Aging

The desire for sexual activity does not usually change as people age. However, men usually require more direct stimulation of genitals and more time to achieve orgasm, with less reliable/strong erections. The intensity of ejaculation usually ↓, and the length of refractory period ↑.

After menopause, women experience vaginal dryness and thinning due to ↓ levels of estrogen and lubrication. They may also have decreased libido and reduced nipple/clitoral/vulvar sensitivity. These conditions can be treated with hormone replacement therapy or vaginal creams.

Differential Diagnosis of Sexual Dysfunctions

Problems with sexual functioning may be due to any of the following:

- Medical conditions: Examples include atherosclerosis (causing erectile dysfunction from vascular occlusion), diabetes (causing erectile dysfunction from vascular changes and peripheral neuropathy), and pelvic adhesions (causing dyspareunia in women).
- Medication side effects: Antihypertensives, anticholinergics, antidepressants (especially selective serotonin reuptake inhibitors [SSRIs]), and antipsychotics may contribute to sexual dysfunctions.
- Depression.
- Substance use.
- Abnormal levels of gonadal hormones:
  - **Estrogen:** ↓ levels after menopause cause vaginal dryness and thinning in women (without affecting desire).

WARDS TIP

Alcohol and marijuana enhance sexual desire by suppressing inhibitions. However, long-term alcohol use decreases sexual desire. Cocaine and amphetamines enhance libido by stimulating dopamine receptors. Narcotics inhibit libido.

- **Testosterone:** Promotes libido (desire) in both men and women.
- **Progesterone:** May inhibit libido in both men and women by blocking androgen receptors; found in oral contraceptives, hormone replacement therapy, and, occasionally, treatments for prostate cancer.
- Presence of a sexual dysfunction (see below).

Sexual Dysfunctions

Sexual dysfunctions are problems involving any stage of the sexual response cycle. They all share the following *Diagnostic and Statistical Manual of Mental Disorders*, 5th ed. (DSM-5) criteria:

- The disorder causes clinically significant distress.
- The dysfunction is not better explained by a nonsexual mental disorder, as a consequence of severe relationship distress or other stressors, and not attributable to the effects of a substance/medication or another medical condition.

Mr. Jones is a 58-year-old married man with a history of major depressive disorder who arrives at your outpatient clinic for a yearly follow-up visit. He complains of recent marital problems with his wife of 30 years. He is being treated with an SSRI, and his depressive symptoms have been stable for over 3 years on his current dose. Upon further questioning, he reveals that he has been having sex with his wife less often than usual, "only once or twice a month." He states that this is a marked decrease since his last visit with you. He feels that lately they have been arguing more and feels that their decrease in sexual activity has adversely affected their relationship. He also reports a mild decrease in his energy.

Mr. Jones denies having urges to masturbate in the times between sexual intercourse with his wife. He also denies having any affairs, laughing nervously while saying, "I can barely satisfy my own wife." He appears sad and states that he is beginning to feel "down" about this. When he does have sex, he reports that it is initiated by his wife, and he is initially reluctant to engage in sexual activity. However, once he does, he denies any problems with having or sustaining an erection and denies any difficulties in reaching orgasm. Mr. Jones reports that he drinks two or three drinks per day on the weekends, and he does not use any recreational drugs.

What is his most likely diagnosis? What other considerations should be made?

The patient's most likely diagnosis is male hypoactive sexual desire disorder. Although decreased sexual interest is more prevalent in women, it should not be overlooked in men. As this clinical case shows, the patient does not seem to fantasize or desire sexual activity despite prior history of doing so. He appears distressed by this and reports that it is causing interpersonal dysfunction. Although his depression has remained stable during the past 3 years and the patient does not report symptoms that would suggest a current depressive episode, his sexual complaints and fatigue symptoms might suggest a relapse of depressive symptoms and should be monitored closely. It is also very important to consider if his treatment with an SSRI is affecting his sexual functioning.

KEY FACT

Dopamine enhances libido. Serotonin inhibits sexual function.

WARDS TIP

Causes of sexual dysfunctions may be physiological or psychological. Psychological causes of sexual dysfunctions are often comorbid with other psychiatric disorders, such as depression or anxiety.

WARDS TIP

Problems with sexual desire may be due to stress, relationship difficulties or conflict, poor self-esteem, or unconscious fears about sex.

> ### What should you consider in the initial management of this patient's complaints?
>
> His initial management should consist of a thorough history, a physical examination, and laboratory tests (complete metabolic profile, testosterone levels, thyroid-stimulating hormone levels) that might rule out medical (e.g., endocrine) abnormalities. If another medical disorder, mental disorder, or substance is believed responsible, treatment considerations should include outpatient psychotherapy, sex therapy, cognitive-behavioral therapy, or group therapy.

- **Male hypoactive sexual desire disorder:** Absence or deficiency of sexual thoughts, desire, or fantasies for >6 months (occurs in <2% of men).
- **Female sexual interest/arousal disorder:** Absence or reduced sexual interest, thoughts/fantasies, initiation of sex, sexual excitement/pleasure, sexual arousal, and/or genital/nongenital sensations during sex for >6 months (unclear prevalence of DSM-5 disorder, but low sexual desire in up to 26–43% of women).
- **Erectile disorder:** Marked difficulty obtaining or maintaining an erection, or marked decreased in erectile rigidity for >6 months. Commonly referred to as *erectile dysfunction (ED)* or *impotence*. May be *lifelong* (never had one) or *acquired* (after previous ability to maintain erections).
- **Premature (early) ejaculation:** Recurrent pattern of ejaculation during sex within 1 minute and before the individual wishes it for >6 months. Up to 30% of men report concerns about how rapidly they ejaculate.
- **Female orgasmic disorder:** Marked delay in/infrequency/absence/reduced intensity of orgasm for >6 months. The prevalence ranges from 10 to 42%.
- **Delayed ejaculation:** Marked delay in/infrequency/absence of ejaculation for >6 months. Estimated prevalence likely <1%.
- **Genito-pelvic pain/penetration disorder:** Persistent or recurrent difficulties in one of the following: vaginal penetration during intercourse, marked vulvovaginal or pelvic pain during intercourse or penetration, marked anticipatory fear or anxiety about vulvovaginal or pelvic pain, or marked tensing or tightening of pelvic floor muscles during attempted vaginal penetration for >6 months. Prevalence unknown but up to 15% of American women complain of pain during intercourse. Controversial whether prior sexual/physical abuse or religious orthodoxy predispose.

Treatment of Sexual Disorders

SEX THERAPY

Sex therapy utilizes the concept of the marital unit, rather than the individual, as the target of therapy. Couples meet with a therapist together in sessions to identify and discuss their sexual problems. The therapist recommends sexual exercises for the couple to attempt at home; activities initially focus on heightening sensory awareness (sensate focus exercises) and progressively incorporate ↑ levels of sexual contact. Treatment is short term. This therapy is most useful when no other psychopathology is involved.

COGNITIVE-BEHAVIORAL THERAPY

Cognitive-behavioral therapy approaches sexual dysfunction as a learned maladaptive behavior. It utilizes traditional therapies such as cognitive restructuring, partner communication training, systematic desensitization, and exposure, where patients are progressively exposed to increasing levels of stimuli that provoke their anxiety. Eventually, patients are able to respond appropriately to the stimuli. Other forms of therapy may include muscle relaxation techniques, assertiveness training, and prescribed sexual exercises to try at home. It is also a short-term therapy.

HYPNOSIS

Most often used adjunctively with other therapies. More useful if anxiety is present.

GROUP THERAPY

May be used as a primary or adjunctive therapy.

ANALYTICALLY ORIENTED (PSYCHODYNAMIC) PSYCHOTHERAPY

Individual, long-term therapy that focuses on feelings, past relationships (including familial), fears, fantasies, dreams, and interpersonal problems that may be contributing to sexual disorder.

PHARMACOLOGIC TREATMENT

- **Erectile disorder:** Phosphodiesterase-5 inhibitors (e.g., sildenafil) are given orally which enhance blood flow to the penis; they require psychological or physical stimulation to achieve an erection. Alprostadil, either injected into the corpora cavernosa or transurethral, acts locally; it produces an erection within 2–3 minutes and works in the absence of sexual stimulation.
- **Premature ejaculation:** SSRIs and tricyclic antidepressants (TCAs) prolong the time from stimulation to orgasm.
- **Male hypoactive sexual desire disorder/Female sexual interest/arousal disorder:** Testosterone is used as replacement therapy for men with low levels. Low doses may also improve libido in women, especially in postmenopausal women. Low-dose vaginal estrogen replacement may improve vaginal dryness and atrophy in postmenopausal women.

MECHANICAL THERAPIES

- **Erectile disorder:** Vacuum-assisted erection devices, occlusive rings, or surgical insertion of semirigid or inflatable tubes into the corpora cavernosa (used only for end-stage impotence).
- **Female orgasmic disorder:** Directed masturbation (education and self-awareness exercises to reach orgasm through self-stimulation).
- **Premature ejaculation:**
  - The *squeeze technique* is used to ↑ the threshold of excitability. When the man is excited to near ejaculation, he or his sexual partner is instructed to squeeze the glans of his penis in order to prevent ejaculation. Gradually, he gains awareness about his sexual sensations and learns to achieve greater ejaculatory control.

- The *stop-start technique* involves cessation of all penile stimulation when the man is near ejaculation. This technique functions in the same manner as the squeeze technique.
- **Genito-pelvic pain/penetration disorder:** Gradual desensitization to achieve intercourse, starting with muscle relaxation techniques, progressing to erotic massage, and finally achieving sexual intercourse.

Gender Dysphoria

Gender dysphoria is commonly referred to as *gender identity disorder, transgender,* or *transsexuality.* Individuals have **distress** accompanying the incongruence between their expressed gender and assigned gender. They may dress as the opposite sex, take sex hormones, or undergo sex change operations.

Cross-gender behaviors in children with this disorder often begin around age 3, the time when gender identity is established. Adults in whom the disorder is first diagnosed usually have experienced some feelings of gender discomfort from early childhood, although the history is not always clear.

Gender dysphoria is often associated with psychological comorbidities such as major depression, anxiety disorders, and suicide.

DIAGNOSIS AND DSM-5 CRITERIA

A. **At least two of the following:**
   1. A marked incongruence between one's experienced gender and primary/secondary sex characteristics
   2. A strong desire to be rid of one's primary/secondary sex characteristics because of the above
   3. A strong desire for the primary/secondary sex characteristics of the other gender
   4. A strong desire to be of the other gender
   5. A strong desire to be treated as the other gender
   6. A strong conviction that one has the typical feelings/reactions of the other gender
B. Clinically significant distress or impairment in functioning

TREATMENT

Therapy and family involvement for younger patients; surgical sex reassignment after living 1 year in the desired gender role and after 1 year of continuous hormone therapy.

Paraphilias

Paraphilic disorders are characterized by engagement in unusual sexual activities and/or preoccupation with unusual sexual urges or fantasies for at least 6 months that either are acted on with a nonconsenting person, or cause significant distress or impairment in functioning. Paraphilic fantasies alone are not considered disorders unless they are intense, recurrent, and interfere with daily life; occasional fantasies are considered normal components of sexuality (even if unusual).

KEY FACT

Transsexuals identify themselves more with the opposite (of their assigned) gender and commonly undergo surgery to physically appear like the opposite (of their assigned) gender.

Only a small percentage of people suffer from paraphilic disorders. Most paraphilic disorders occur almost exclusively in men, but sadism, masochism, and pedophilia may also occur in women. Voyeuristic and pedophilic disorders are the most common paraphilic disorders.

EXAMPLES OF PARAPHILIC DISORDERS

- **Pedophilic disorder:** Sexual fantasies/urges/behaviors involving sexual acts with prepubescent children (age 13 years or younger). DSM-5 specifies that the person is at least age 16 and at least 5 years older than the child.
- **Frotteuristic disorder:** Sexual arousal from touching or rubbing against a nonconsenting person.
- **Voyeuristic disorder:** Sexual arousal from observing an unsuspecting nude, or disrobing individual (often with binoculars).
- **Exhibitionistic disorder:** Sexual arousal from exposure of one's genitals to an unsuspecting person.
- **Sexual masochism disorder:** Sexual arousal from the act of being humiliated, beaten, bound, or made to suffer.
- **Sexual sadism disorder:** Sexual arousal from the physical or psychological suffering of another person.
- **Fetishistic disorder:** Sexual arousal from either the use of nonliving objects (e.g., shoes or pantyhose) or nongenital body parts.
- **Transvestic disorder:** Sexual arousal from cross-dressing (e.g., wearing women's clothing such as underwear).

Course and Prognosis

- *Poor prognostic factors* are having multiple paraphilias, early age of onset, comorbid substance use, high frequency of behavior, and referral by law enforcement agencies (i.e., after an arrest).
- *Good prognostic factors* are having only one paraphilia, self-referral for treatment, sense of guilt associated with the behavior, and history of otherwise normal sexual activity in addition to the paraphilia.

Treatment

- Difficult to treat
- Psychotropic medication if associated with a comorbid psychiatric illness
- Although controversial, antiandrogens, long-acting gonadotropin-releasing hormones, SSRIs, and naltrexone have been used to decrease sex drive and fantasies
- Cognitive-behavioral therapy can be used to disrupt learned patterns and modify behavior
- Social skills training
- 12-step programs
- Group therapy
- Insight-oriented therapy has been used with questionable benefit

KEY FACT

The three most common types of paraphilia: pedophilia, voyeurism, exhibitionism.

KEY FACT

Patients often have more than one paraphilia.

KEY FACT

An example of fetishistic disorder is a man being primarily sexually aroused by women's shoes causing significant distress and marital problems.

KEY FACT

An example of transvestic disorder is a person being sexually aroused by dressing up as a member of the opposite gender. This does *not* mean they are homosexual.

KEY FACT

Most rape offenders are relatives of the victim.

CHAPTER 17

PSYCHOTHERAPIES

Psychoanalysis and Related Therapies   180

Freud's Theories of the Mind   180

    TOPOGRAPHIC THEORY   180

    STRUCTURAL THEORY   180

Defense Mechanisms   180

    MATURE DEFENSES   181

    NEUROTIC DEFENSES   181

    IMMATURE DEFENSES   182

    OTHER DEFENSE MECHANISMS   182

Psychoanalysis   182

    IMPORTANT CONCEPTS AND TECHNIQUES USED IN PSYCHOANALYSIS   183

    PSYCHOANALYSIS-RELATED THERAPIES   183

Behavioral Therapy   184

    LEARNING THEORY   184

    CONDITIONING   184

    BEHAVIORAL THERAPY TECHNIQUES (DECONDITIONING) 184

Cognitive Therapy   185

    CLINICAL EXAMPLE OF THE COGNITIVE THEORY OF DEPRESSION   185

Cognitive-Behavioral Therapy (CBT)   185

Dialectical Behavioral Therapy (DBT)   186

Group Therapy   186

Family Therapy   187

Couples Therapy   187

It is common to combine psychotherapy with medications. *Split treatment* describes the arrangement where a psychiatrist prescribes medication and someone else provides therapy; in these cases the psychiatrist and therapist should regularly communicate regarding the patient's treatment.

Psychoanalysis and Related Therapies

Psychoanalysis and its related therapies are derived from Sigmund Freud's psychoanalytic theories of the mind. Freud proposed that behaviors, or symptoms, result from *unconscious* mental processes, including defense mechanisms and conflicts between one's ego, id, superego, and external reality. Since the time of Freud, many other psychoanalytic theories have been developed. Influential theorists have included Melanie Klein, Heinz Kohut, Michael Balint, Margaret Mahler, and others.

Examples of psychoanalytic therapies include:
- Psychoanalysis
- Psychoanalytically oriented psychotherapy
- Brief dynamic therapy
- Interpersonal therapy

Freud's Theories of the Mind

TOPOGRAPHIC THEORY

1. **Unconscious:** Includes repressed thoughts that are out of one's awareness; involves *primary process* thinking (primitive, pleasure-seeking urges with no regard to logic or time, prominent in children and psychosis). Thoughts and ideas may be repressed into the unconscious because they are embarrassing, shameful, or otherwise too painful.
2. **Preconscious:** Contains memories that are easy to bring into awareness, but not unless consciously retrieved.
3. **Conscious:** Involves current thoughts and secondary process thinking (logical, organized, mature, and can delay gratification).

STRUCTURAL THEORY

1. **Id:** Unconscious; involves instinctual sexual/aggressive urges and primary process thinking.
2. **Superego:** Moral conscience and ego ideal (inner image of oneself that one wants to become).
3. **Ego:** Serves as a mediator between the id, superego, and external environment and seeks to develop satisfying interpersonal relationships; uses *defense mechanisms* (see below) to control instinctual urges and distinguishes fantasy from reality using *reality testing*. Problems with reality testing occur in psychotic individuals.

Defense Mechanisms

Defense mechanisms are used by the ego to protect oneself and relieve anxiety by keeping conflicts out of awareness. They are (mostly) *unconscious* processes that are normal and healthy if mature and when used in moderation (i.e., adaptive), but may be unhealthy and seen in some psychiatric disorders when used excessively (i.e., maladaptive).

Defense mechanisms are often classified hierarchically. **Mature** defense mechanisms are healthy and adaptive, and they are seen in normal adults. **Neurotic** defenses are encountered in obsessive-compulsive patients, patients with other anxiety disorders, and adults under stress. **Immature** defenses are seen in children, adolescents, psychotic patients, and some nonpsychotic patients, such as patients with severe personality disorders. They are the most primitive defense mechanisms.

MATURE DEFENSES

A former street thug becomes a social worker to help reform kids in gangs. *What is the defense mechanism?* Sublimation—the channeling of destructive impulses to create something constructive.

Mature ego defenses are commonly found in healthy, high-functioning adults. These defenses often help people integrate conflicting emotions and thoughts.

1. **Altruism:** Performing acts that benefit others in order to vicariously experience pleasure. (*Clinical example:* A patient's child recently died from ovarian cancer. As part of the grieving process, the patient donates money to help raise community awareness about the symptoms of ovarian cancer so other patients could potentially benefit from early intervention.)
2. **Humor:** Expressing (usually) unpleasant or uncomfortable feelings without causing discomfort to self or others.
3. **Sublimation:** Satisfying socially objectionable impulses in an acceptable manner (thus *channeling* them rather than *preventing* them). (*Clinical example:* Person with unconscious urges to physically control others becomes a prison guard.)
4. **Suppression:** Purposely ignoring an unacceptable impulse or emotion in order to diminish discomfort and accomplish a task. (*Clinical example:* Nurse who feels nauseated by an infected wound puts aside feelings of disgust to clean wound and provide necessary patient care.)

> **KEY FACT**
>
> Suppression, as a defense mechanism, is a *conscious* process that involves avoiding paying attention to a particular emotion. Therefore, it is not an unconscious process.

NEUROTIC DEFENSES

A man buys himself an expensive new watch and tells his friends that he needed it because his old one was not reliable enough and he needs to make sure to get to his appointments on time. *Think: Rationalization.*

1. **Controlling:** Regulating situations and events of external environment to relieve anxiety.
2. **Displacement:** Shifting emotions from an undesirable situation to one that is personally tolerable. (*Clinical example:* Student who is angry with his mother talks back to his teacher the next day and refuses to obey her instructions.)

3. **Intellectualization:** Avoiding negative feelings by excessive use of intellectual functions and by focusing on irrelevant details. (*Clinical example:* Physician dying from colon cancer describes the pathophysiology of his disease in detail to his 12-year-old son.)

4. **Isolation of affect:** Unconsciously limiting the experience of feelings or emotions associated with a stressful life event in order to avoid anxiety. (*Clinical example:* Woman describes the recent death of her beloved husband without emotion.)

5. **Rationalization:** Explanations of an event in order to justify outcomes or behaviors and to make them acceptable. (*Clinical example:* "My boss fired me today because she's not meeting her quotas, not because I haven't done a good job.")

6. **Reaction formation:** Doing the opposite of an unacceptable impulse. (*Clinical example:* Man who is in love with his married coworker insults her.)

7. **Repression:** Preventing a thought or feeling from entering consciousness. (Repression is unconscious, whereas suppression is a conscious act.)

IMMATURE DEFENSES

1. **Acting out:** Giving in to an impulse, even if socially inappropriate, in order to avoid the anxiety of suppressing that impulse. (*Clinical example:* Man who has been told his therapist is going on vacation "forgets" his last appointment and skips it.)

2. **Denial:** Not accepting reality that is too painful. (*Clinical example:* Woman who has been scheduled for a breast mass biopsy cancels her appointment because she believes she is healthy.)

3. **Regression:** Performing behaviors from an earlier stage of development in order to avoid tension associated with current phase of development. (*Clinical example:* Woman brings her childhood teddy bear to the hospital when she has to spend the night.)

4. **Projection:** Attributing objectionable thoughts or emotions to others. (*Clinical example:* Husband who is attracted to other women believes his wife is having an affair.)

OTHER DEFENSE MECHANISMS

1. **Splitting:** Labeling people as all good or all bad (often seen in borderline personality disorder). (*Clinical example:* Woman who tells her doctor, "You and the nurses are the only people who understand me; all the other doctors are mean and impatient.")

2. **Undoing:** Attempting to reverse a situation by adopting a new behavior. (*Clinical example:* Man who has had a brief fantasy of killing his wife by sabotaging her car takes the car in for a complete checkup.)

Psychoanalysis

The goal of psychoanalysis is to resolve *unconscious conflicts* by bringing repressed experiences and feelings into awareness and integrating them into the patient's conscious experience. Psychoanalysis is therefore considered *insight oriented.* Patients best suited for psychoanalysis have the following characteristics: not psychotic, intelligent, and stable in relationships and daily living. Treatment is usually 3–5 days per week for many years. During therapy sessions, the patient usually lies on a couch with the therapist seated out of view.

To become an analyst, individuals (MDs, PhDs, PsyDs, and MSWs) must complete training at a psychoanalytic institute. In addition to attending seminars and treating patients under supervision, the training requires that they receive their own analysis.

Psychoanalysis can be useful in the treatment of:
- Clusters B and C personality disorders
- Anxiety disorders
- Problems coping with life events
- Sexual disorders
- Persistent depressive disorder

IMPORTANT CONCEPTS AND TECHNIQUES USED IN PSYCHOANALYSIS

- **Free association:** The patient is asked to say whatever comes into his or her mind during therapy sessions. The purpose is to bring forth thoughts and feelings from the unconscious so that the therapist may interpret them.
- **Dream interpretation:** Dreams are seen to represent conflict between urges and fears. Interpretation of dreams by the psychoanalyst is used to help achieve therapeutic goals.
- **Therapeutic alliance:** This is the bond between the therapist and the patient, who work together toward a therapeutic goal.
- **Transference:** Projection of unconscious feelings regarding important figures in the patient's life onto the therapist. Interpretation of transference is used to help the patient gain insight and resolve unconscious conflict.
- **Countertransference:** Projection of unconscious feelings about important figures in the therapist's life onto the patient. The therapist must remain aware of countertransference issues, as they may interfere with his or her objectivity.

> **KEY FACT**
>
> An example of transference would be when a patient who has repressed feelings of abandonment by her father becomes angry when her therapist is late for the appointment.

PSYCHOANALYSIS-RELATED THERAPIES

Examples of psychoanalysis-related therapies include:

1. **Psychoanalytically oriented psychotherapy** and **brief dynamic psychotherapy:** These employ similar techniques and theories as psychoanalysis, but they are less frequent, less intense, usually briefer (weekly sessions for 6 months to several years), and involve face-to-face sessions between the therapist and patient (no couch).
2. **Interpersonal therapy:** Focuses on development of social skills to help treat certain psychiatric disorders. Treatment is short (once-weekly sessions for several months). The idea is to improve interpersonal relations. Sessions focus on reassurance, clarification of emotions, improving interpersonal communication, and testing perceptions.
3. **Supportive psychotherapy:** Purpose is to help patient feel safe during a difficult time and help to build up the patient's healthy defenses. Treatment is not insight oriented but instead focuses on empathy, understanding, and education. Supportive therapy is commonly used as adjunctive treatment in even the most severe mental disorders.

Behavioral Therapy

Behavioral therapy, pioneered by B. F. Skinner, seeks to treat psychiatric disorders by helping patients change behaviors that contribute to their symptoms. It can be used to extinguish maladaptive behaviors (such as phobic avoidance, compulsions, etc.) by replacing them with healthy alternatives. The time course is usually brief, and it is usually combined with cognitive therapy as CBT.

LEARNING THEORY

Behavioral therapy is based on **learning theory,** which states that behaviors are learned by *conditioning* and can similarly be unlearned by *deconditioning*.

CONDITIONING

- **Classical conditioning:** A stimulus can evoke a conditioned response. (*Example:* Pavlov's dog would salivate when hearing a bell because the dog had learned that bells were always followed by food.)
- **Operant conditioning:** Behaviors can be learned when followed by positive or negative *reinforcement*. (*Example:* Skinner box—a rat presses a lever by accident and receives food; eventually, it learns to press the lever for food [trial-and-error learning].)

BEHAVIORAL THERAPY TECHNIQUES (DECONDITIONING)

- **Systematic desensitization:** The patient performs relaxation techniques while being exposed to increasing doses of an anxiety-provoking stimulus. Gradually, he or she learns to associate the stimulus with a state of relaxation. Commonly used to treat phobic disorders. (*Example:* A patient who has a fear of spiders is first shown a photograph of a spider, followed by exposure to a stuffed toy spider, then a videotape of a spider, and finally a live spider. At each step, the patient learns to relax while exposed to an increasing dose of the phobia.)
- **Flooding and implosion:** Through habituation, the patient is confronted with a real (flooding) or imagined (implosion) anxiety-provoking stimulus and not allowed to withdraw from it until he or she feels calm and in control. Relaxation exercises are used to help the patient tolerate the stimulus. Less commonly (than systematic desensitization) used to treat phobic disorders. (*Example:* A patient who has a fear of flying is made to fly in an airplane [flooding] or imagine flying [implosion].)
- **Aversion therapy:** A negative stimulus (such as an electric shock) is repeatedly paired with a specific behavior to create an unpleasant response. Used to treat addictions or paraphilias. (*Example:* An alcoholic patient is prescribed Antabuse, which makes him ill every time he drinks alcohol.)
- **Token economy:** Rewards are given after specific behaviors to positively reinforce them. Commonly used to encourage showering, shaving, and other positive behaviors in disorganized patients or individuals on addiction rehabilitation units.
- **Biofeedback:** Physiological data (such as heart rate and blood pressure measurements) are given to patients as they try to mentally control physiological states. Can be used to treat anxiety disorders, migraines, hypertension, chronic pain, asthma, and incontinence. (*Example:* A patient is given her heart rate and blood pressure measurements during a migraine while being instructed to mentally control visceral changes that affect her pain.)

KEY FACT

Positive reinforcement: Giving a reward for a desired behavior.

KEY FACT

Negative reinforcement: Encouraging a behavior by removing an aversive stimulus. Punishment, in contrast, is an aversive response to a behavior. Punishment is *not* negative reinforcement.

Cognitive Therapy

Cognitive therapy, pioneered by Aaron T. Beck, seeks to correct faulty assumptions and negative feelings that exacerbate psychiatric symptoms. The patient is taught to identify maladaptive thoughts and replace them with positive ones. Most commonly used to treat depressive and anxiety disorders, and it is usually combined with behavioral therapy as CBT. May also be used for paranoid personality disorder, obsessive-compulsive disorder, somatic symptom disorders, and eating disorders. Cognitive therapy can be as effective as medication.

CLINICAL EXAMPLE OF THE COGNITIVE THEORY OF DEPRESSION

- **Cognitive distortions,** also known as **faulty assumptions** (*Example:* If I were smart, I would do well on tests. I must not be smart since I received average grades this semester.)
- **Negative thoughts** (*Example:* I am stupid. I will never amount to anything worthwhile. Nobody likes a worthless person.)

Cognitive-Behavioral Therapy (CBT)

CBT combines theories and approaches from cognitive therapy and behavior therapy. Treatment follows a protocol or manual with homework assignments between therapy sessions. During therapy sessions, the patient and therapist set an **agenda,** review homework, and challenge cognitive distortions. The patients learn how their feelings and behavior are influenced by their thoughts. Treatment is usually brief and may last from 6 weeks to 6 months. Research has shown that CBT is effective for many psychiatric illnesses, including depression, anxiety disorders, schizophrenia, and substance use disorders.

KEY FACT

Biofeedback used to treat a wide scope of clinical conditions including agoraphobia, fecal incontinence, tension headache, and hypertension.

WARDS TIP

CBT focuses on a patient's current symptoms and problems by examining the connection between thoughts, feelings, and behaviors.

Mrs. Ramos is a 22-year-old college student who is hospitalized after she tried to kill herself by taking an overdose of fluoxetine. This is her fifth overdose, and all have been in response to perceived rejections. She often feels "empty inside" and reports that she has had many intense relationships that have ended abruptly. She reports that she has been married for 1 year but fights constantly with her husband because of suspicions that he is unfaithful. Her husband denies these allegations and reports that he is tired of her outbursts, explaining that she yells at him and has become physically abusive. He has threatened to divorce her if these behaviors continue. During your evaluation, you notice multiple healed scars over her forearms, and she admits to self-harm behavior by cutting and burning herself because, "When I get angry, it helps me feel better."

During her hospitalization, you notice that her mood has improved and that she has become close to other patients. She says, "They are like family." Although you have seen her only twice, she thinks you are "a great doctor," unlike the psychiatrists who have treated her in the past, who have all been "idiots." You call her outpatient therapist, who confirms that she has been diagnosed with borderline personality disorder.

What are the recommended psychotherapeutic modalities for this patient?

Dialectical behavioral therapy (DBT) and psychoanalytic/psychodynamic therapy have shown to be effective treatments in randomized controlled trials for borderline personality disorder. DBT is a form of cognitive-behavioral therapy that is effective in reducing the urges to engage in self-harm behavior and leads to fewer hospital days. Although the efficacy of couples therapy in borderline patients has been debated, it might be considered in this case.

What special considerations should be taken into account when engaging in psychotherapy?

The psychotherapist should always be aware of positive or negative countertransference developed toward the patient. Frequent discussion and counseling with colleagues is useful. Borderline patients are challenging to treat due to their intense emotions, impulsivity, and anger.

What particular defense mechanism is exhibited by Mrs. Ramos?

Mrs. Ramos exhibits splitting as evidenced by her extreme dichotomous thinking in expressing that you are a "great" psychiatrist, whereas other psychiatrists who have treated her in the past are "idiots."

Dialectical Behavioral Therapy (DBT)

DBT was developed by Marsha Linehan, and its effectiveness has been demonstrated in research trials. Once-weekly individual and group treatment can effectively diminish the self-destructive behaviors and hospitalizations of patients with borderline personality disorder. It incorporates cognitive and supportive techniques, along with the "mindfulness" derived from traditional Buddhist practice. DBT has demonstrated effectiveness in patients with borderline personality disorders.

Group Therapy

- Three or more patients with a similar problem or pathology meet together with a therapist for group sessions. Many of the psychotherapeutic techniques already reviewed are used, including behavioral, cognitive, and supportive.
- Certain groups are *peer led* (including 12-step groups like Alcoholics Anonymous) and do not have a therapist present to facilitate the group. These groups meet to discuss problems, share feelings, and provide support to each other.
- Group therapy is especially useful in the treatment of substance use disorders, adjustment disorders, and personality disorders. Advantages of group therapy over individual therapy include:
  - Patients get immediate feedback and support from their peers.
  - Patients gain insight into their own condition by listening to others with similar problems.
  - If a therapist is present, there is an opportunity to observe interactions between others who may be eliciting a variety of transferences.

Family Therapy

Family therapy is useful as an adjunctive treatment in many psychiatric conditions because:

1. An individual's problems usually affect the entire family. He or she may be viewed differently and treated differently after the development of psychopathology, and new tensions and conflicts within the family may arise.
2. Psychopathology may arise or worsen due to dysfunction within the family unit. These conditions are most effectively treated with the entire family present.

The goals of family therapy are to reduce conflict, help members understand each other's needs (*mutual accommodation*), and help the family unit cope with internally destructive forces. **Boundaries** between family members may be too rigid or too permeable, and **"triangles"** may result when two family members form an alliance against a third member. The therapist may assist in correcting these problems. (*Example of boundaries that may be too permeable*: A mother and daughter smoke marijuana together and share intimate details about their sexual activities.) Family therapy is especially useful in treating schizophrenia and anorexia in adolescents.

Couples Therapy

Couples therapy is useful in the treatment of conflicts, sexual problems, and communication problems within the context of an intimate relationship. The therapist sees the couple together (**conjoint therapy**), but they may also be seen separately (**concurrent therapy**). In addition, each person may have a separate therapist and be seen individually (**collaborative therapy**). In the treatment of sexual problems, two therapists may see the couple together (**four-way therapy**). Relative contraindications include lack of motivation by one or both spouses and severe illness in one of the spouses (e.g., schizophrenia).

NOTES

CHAPTER 18

PSYCHOPHARMACOLOGY

Side Effects in a Nutshell	190
Antidepressants	191
SELECTIVE SEROTONIN REUPTAKE INHIBITORS	191
MISCELLANEOUS ANTIDEPRESSANTS	192
HETEROCYCLIC ANTIDEPRESSANTS: TCAs	193
TRICYCLIC ANTIDEPRESSANTS	194
TETRACYCLIC ANTIDEPRESSANTS	194
MONOAMINE OXIDASE INHIBITORS	195
Antidepressant Use in Other Disorders	195
Antipsychotics	196
TYPICAL (FIRST-GENERATION) ANTIPSYCHOTICS	196
ATYPICAL (SECOND-GENERATION) ANTIPSYCHOTICS	199
Mood Stabilizers	200
LITHIUM	200
Anticonvulsants	201
CARBAMAZEPINE (TEGRETOL)	201
VALPROIC ACID (DEPAKOTE AND DEPAKENE)	202
Anxiolytics/Hypnotics	202
BENZODIAZEPINES	203

NON-BDZ HYPNOTICS	204
NON-BDZ ANXIOLYTICS	204
Psychostimulants	204
Cognitive Enhancers	205
ACETYLCHOLINESTERASE INHIBITORS	205
NMDA (GLUTAMATE) RECEPTOR ANTAGONIST	205
Summary of Medications That May Cause Psychiatric Symptoms	205
PSYCHOSIS	205
AGITATION/CONFUSION/DELIRIUM	206
DEPRESSION	206
ANXIETY	206
SEDATION/POOR CONCENTRATION	206
SELECTED MEDICATIONS	206
Other Treatments	206
ELECTROCONVULSIVE THERAPY (ECT)	206
DEEP BRAIN STIMULATION (DBS)	207
REPETITIVE TRANSCRANIAL MAGNETIC STIMULATION (rTMS)	207
LIGHT THERAPY	207

Side Effects in a Nutshell

1. **HAM side effects** (*antiHistamine*—sedation, weight gain; *antiAdrenergic*—hypotension; *antiMuscarinic*—dry mouth, blurred vision, urinary retention, constipation). Found in tricyclic antidepressants (TCAs) and low-potency antipsychotics.
2. **Serotonin syndrome:** Confusion, flushing, diaphoresis, tremor, myoclonic jerks, hyperthermia, hypertonicity, rhabdomyolysis, renal failure, and death.
   - Occurs when there is too much serotonin, classically when selective serotonin reuptake inhibitors (SSRIs) and monoamine oxidase inhibitors (MAOIs) are combined.
   - Treatment: Stop medications, supportive care.
3. **Hypertensive crisis:** Caused by a buildup of stored catecholamines; caused by the combination of MAOIs with tyramine-rich foods (e.g., red wine, cheese, chicken liver, cured meats) or with sympathomimetics.
4. **Extrapyramidal side effects (EPS):** *Parkinsonism*—masklike face, cogwheel rigidity, bradykinesia, pill-rolling tremor; *akathisia*—restlessness, need to move, and agitation; *dystonia*—sustained, painful contraction of muscles of neck, tongue, eyes, diaphragm.
   - Occur with high-potency, typical (first generation) antipsychotics
   - Reversible
   - Occur within *hours to days* of starting medications or increasing doses
   - In rare cases can be life threatening (e.g., dystonia of the diaphragm causing asphyxiation)
5. **Hyperprolactinemia:** Occurs with high-potency, typical (first generation) antipsychotics and risperidone.
6. **Tardive dyskinesia (TD):** Choreoathetoid muscle movements, usually of the mouth and tongue (can affect extremities, as well).
   - Occurs after *years* of antipsychotic use (more likely with high-potency, first-generation antipsychotics)
   - Usually is irreversible
7. **Neuroleptic malignant syndrome: Mental status changes,** fever, tachycardia, hypertension, tremor, elevated creatine phosphokinase (CPK), "lead pipe" rigidity.
   - Can be caused by any antipsychotic after a short or long time (↑ with high-potency, typical antipsychotics)
   - A medical emergency with up to a 20% mortality rate
8. **Drug interactions:** *Cytochrome P450* is a group of enzymes in the liver that metabolizes many common drugs, including psychiatric medications.
   - Some medications *induce* the system, in other words the system metabolizes medications faster—drug levels *decrease*.
   - Some medications *inhibit* the system, in other words the system metabolizes medications more slowly—drug levels *increase*.
   - Common cytochrome P450 enzymes important in metabolizing psychiatric medications include CYP3A4, CYP2D6, CYP1A2, CYP2C9, CYP2C19.
   - Important CYP450 *inducers* include:
     - Tobacco (1A2)
     - Carbamazepine (1A2, 2C9, 3A4)
     - Barbiturates (2C9)
     - St. John's wort (2C19, 3A4)
   - Important CYP450 *inhibitors* include:
     - Fluvoxamine (1A2, 2C19, 3A4)
     - Fluoxetine (2C19, 2C9, 2D6)
     - Paroxetine (2D6)

KEY FACT

The first-line treatment for extrapyramidal symptoms caused by antipsychotics is benztropine (Cogentin).

KEY FACT

Keeping the "kinesias" (impairment of body function) straight:
- Tardive dyskinesia is characterized by grimacing and tongue protrusion.
- Acute dystonia is characterized by twisting and abnormal postures.
- Akathisia is characterized by the inability to sit still.
- Bradykinesia is characterized by ↓ or slow body movement.

KEY FACT

Constipation is a common side effect of anticholinergic medications.

KEY FACT

Anticholinergic medications exacerbate neurocognitive disorders (dementias).

- Duloxetine (2D6)
- Sertraline (2D6)

Antidepressants

- The major categories of antidepressants are:
  - SSRIs
  - Heterocyclic antidepressants, including TCAs and tetracyclic antidepressants
  - MAOIs
  - Miscellaneous antidepressants
- All antidepressants have similar response rates in treating major depression but differ in safety and side-effect profiles.
- Approximately 60–70% of patients with major depression will respond to an antidepressant medication.
- Most antidepressants require a trial of at least 3–4 weeks for any effect, with some people requiring as little as 1–2 weeks and some 6–8 weeks for significant improvement.
- Many antidepressants have a *withdrawal phenomenon*, characterized by dizziness, headaches, nausea, insomnia, and malaise; depending on the dose and half-life, they may need to be tapered.
- Because of their safety and tolerability, SSRIs and related antidepressants have become the most common agents used to treat major depression. However, the choice of a particular medication used for a given patient should be made based on:
  - Patient's particular symptoms
  - Previous treatment responses by the patient or a family member to a particular medication
  - Side-effect profile
  - Comorbid (medical and psychiatric) conditions
  - Risk of suicide via overdose on the medication
  - Cost

SELECTIVE SEROTONIN REUPTAKE INHIBITORS

- SSRIs inhibit presynaptic serotonin pumps that take up serotonin, leading to ↑ availability of serotonin in synaptic clefts. Additionally, SSRIs cause downstream effects increasing brain plasticity—this mechanism has been hypothesized to explain the delay to onset of antidepressant effect.
- Although structural differences are minimal, patients often respond differently (in regards to efficacy and side effects) to different SSRIs.
- Based on their half-lives, most SSRIs can be dosed daily. Fluoxetine has a weekly dosing form available, as well.
- There is no correlation between plasma levels and efficacy or side effects.
- SSRIs are the most commonly prescribed antidepressants due to several distinct advantages:
  - Low incidence of side effects, most of which resolve with time
  - No food restrictions
  - Much safer in overdose
- Examples of SSRIs include:
  - **Fluoxetine (Prozac):**
    - Longest half-life, with active metabolites; therefore, no need to taper
    - Safe in pregnancy, approved for use in children and adolescents
    - Common side effects: insomnia, anxiety, sexual dysfunction
    - Can elevate levels of antipsychotics, leading to ↑ side effects

- **Sertraline (Zoloft):**
    - Higher risk for gastrointestinal (GI) disturbances
    - Very few drug interactions
    - Other common side effects: insomnia, anxiety, sexual dysfunction
- **Paroxetine (Paxil):**
    - Highly protein bound, leading to several drug interactions
    - Common side effects: anticholinergic effects (e.g., sedation, constipation, weight gain) and sexual dysfunction
    - Short half-life leading to *withdrawal phenomena* if not taken consistently
- **Fluvoxamine (Luvox):**
    - Currently approved only for use in obsessive-compulsive disorder (OCD)
    - Common side effects: nausea and vomiting
    - Multiple drug interactions due to CYP inhibition
- **Citalopram (Celexa):**
    - Fewest drug–drug interactions
    - Dose dependent QTc prolongation
- **Escitalopram (Lexapro):**
    - Levo-enantiomer of citalopram; similar efficacy, possibly fewer side effects
    - Dose dependent QTc prolongation

Side Effects

- SSRIs have significantly fewer side effects than TCAs and MAOIs due to serotonin selectivity (they do not act on histamine, adrenergic, or muscarinic receptors).
- They are much safer in overdose. Most side effects occur because of the extensive number of serotonin receptors throughout the body, including the GI tract.
- Many of the side effects of SSRIs resolve within a few days to weeks and include:
    - GI disturbance: Mostly nausea and diarrhea; giving with food can help.
    - Insomnia; also vivid dreams, often resolves over time.
    - Headache.
    - Anorexia, weight loss.
- Other side effects include:
    - Sexual dysfunction (30–40%): ↓ libido, anorgasmia, delayed ejaculation. These may occur weeks to months after taking an SSRI and typically do not resolve.
    - Restlessness: An akathisia-like state.
    - **Serotonin syndrome:** Caused by taking two medications, both of which ↑ serotonin leading to too much serotonin in the brain. An example is triptans (for migraine headaches) used with SSRIs. Serotonin syndrome is characterized by fever, diaphoresis, tachycardia, hypertension, delirium, and neuromuscular excitability (especially hyperreflexia and "electric jolt" limb movements), potentially → death.
    - Hyponatremia: Rare
    - Seizures: Rate of approximately 0.2%, slightly lower than TCAs.

MISCELLANEOUS ANTIDEPRESSANTS

Serotonin-Norepinephrine Reuptake Inhibitors (SNRIs)

- **Venlafaxine (Effexor):**
    - Often used for depression, anxiety disorders like generalized anxiety disorder (GAD), and neuropathic pain

KEY FACT

The FDA has a Black Box Warning for all SSRIs potentially increasing "suicidal thinking and behavior." This warning applies to children and young adults to age 25, but may be accurate for adults as well.

KEY FACT

Serotonin syndrome is common when serotonergic drugs are used with MAOIs. SSRIs should not be used for at least 2 weeks before or after use of an MAOI.

- Low drug interaction potential.
- Extended release (XR form) allows for once-daily dosing.
- Side-effect profile similar to SSRIs, with the exception of ↑ blood pressure (BP) in higher doses; do not use in patients with untreated or labile BP.
- New form, **desvenlafaxine (Pristiq),** is the active metabolite of venlafaxine; it is expensive and without known benefit over venlafaxine.
- **Duloxetine (Cymbalta):**
  - Often used for people with **depression, neuropathic pain,** and in fibromyalgia.
  - Side effects are similar to SSRIs, but more dry mouth and constipation relating to its norepinephrine effects.
  - Hepatotoxicity may be more likely in patients with liver disease or heavy alcohol use.
  - Expensive.

Norepinephrine-Dopamine Reuptake Inhibitors

- **Bupropion (Wellbutrin):**
  - Relative **lack of sexual side effects** as compared to the SSRIs.
  - Some efficacy in treatment of adult ADHD.
  - Effective for smoking cessation.
  - Side effects include ↑ anxiety, as well as ↑ risk of **seizures** and psychosis at high doses.
  - Contraindicated in patients with seizure or active eating disorders, and in those currently on an MAOI.

Serotonin Receptor Antagonists and Agonists

- **Trazodone (Desyrel)** and **Nefazodone (Serzone):**
  - Useful in the treatment of major depression, major depression with anxiety, and **insomnia** (secondary to its sedative effects).
  - They do not have the sexual side effects of SSRIs and do not affect rapid eye movement (REM) sleep.
  - Side effects include nausea, dizziness, orthostatic hypotension, cardiac arrhythmias, **sedation,** and **priapism** (especially with **trazodone**).
  - Because of orthostatic hypotension in higher doses, trazodone is not frequently used solely as an antidepressant. It is commonly used to treat insomnia often when initiating an SSRI (until insomnia improves as the depression resolves).
  - Nefazodone carries a **Black Box Warning** for rare but serious liver failure (1 per 250,000–300,000 people) and is rarely used.

α2-Adrenergic Receptor Antagonists

- **Mirtazapine (Remeron):**
  - Useful in the treatment of **major depression,** especially in patients who have significant weight loss and/or insomnia.
  - Side effects include **sedation, weight gain,** dizziness, tremor, dry mouth, constipation, and (rarely) agranulocytosis.
  - Fewer sexual side effects compared to SSRIs and few drug interactions.

WARDS TIP

SSRIs can ↑ levels of warfarin, requiring ↑ monitoring when starting and stopping these medications.

KEY FACT

Bupropion can lower the seizure threshold. Use with caution in patients with epilepsy and eating disorders.

KEY FACT

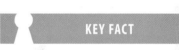

Trazodone causes priapism: tRAZodone will RAISE the bone.

WARDS TIP

Remeron for treating major depression in the elderly—helps with sleep and appetite.

HETEROCYCLIC ANTIDEPRESSANTS

- TCAs inhibit the reuptake of norepinephrine and serotonin, ↑ availability of monoamines in the synapse.
- Because of the long half-lives, most are dosed once daily.

- They are rarely used as first-line agents due to a higher incidence of side effects, titration of dosing, and **lethality in overdose.**

TRICYCLIC ANTIDEPRESSANTS

- **Tertiary amines** (highly anticholinergic/antihistaminergic [more sedating]/ antiadrenergic with a greater lethality in overdose):
    - **Amitriptyline (Elavil):** Useful in chronic pain, migraines, and insomnia.
    - **Imipramine (Tofranil):**
        - Has intramuscular form
        - Useful in **enuresis** and panic disorder
    - **Clomipramine (Anafranil):** Most serotonin-specific, therefore useful in the treatment of **OCD**.
    - **Doxepin (Sinequan):**
        - Useful in treating chronic pain
        - Emerging use as a sleep aid in low doses
- **Secondary amines**—metabolites of tertiary amines (less anticholinergic/ antihistaminic/antiadrenergic):
    - **Nortriptyline (Pamelor, Aventyl):**
        - Least likely to cause orthostatic hypotension
        - Useful therapeutic blood levels
        - Useful in treating chronic pain
    - **Desipramine (Norpramin):**
        - More activating/least sedating
        - Least anticholinergic

TETRACYCLIC ANTIDEPRESSANTS

- **Amoxapine (Asendin):**
    - Metabolite of antipsychotic loxapine
    - May cause EPS and has a similar side-effect profile to typical antipsychotics

Side Effects

- TCAs are *highly* protein bound and lipid soluble, and therefore can interact with other medications that have high protein binding.
- The side effects of TCAs are mostly due to their lack of specificity and interaction with other receptors.
- Antihistaminic properties: Sedation and weight gain.

- Antiadrenergic properties (**cardiovascular** side effects): Orthostatic hypotension, dizziness, reflex tachycardia, arrhythmias (block cardiac sodium channel), and electrocardiographic (ECG) changes (widening QRS, QT, and PR intervals). Avoid in patients with preexisting conduction abnormalities or recent MI.
- Antimuscarinic effects (also called anticholinergic): Dry mouth, constipation, urinary retention, blurred vision, tachycardia, and exacerbation of narrow angle glaucoma.
- Lethal in overdose—must carefully assess the suicide risk when prescribing. Symptoms of overdose include agitation, tremors, ataxia, arrhythmias, delirium, hypoventilation from central nervous system (CNS) depression, myoclonus, hyperreflexia, seizures, and coma.

- Seizures: Occur at a rate of about 0.4%, more common at higher plasma levels and with clomipramine and tetracyclics.
- Serotonergic effects: Erectile/ejaculatory dysfunction in males, anorgasmia in females.

MONOAMINE OXIDASE INHIBITORS

- MAOIs prevent the inactivation of biogenic amines such as *norepinephrine*, *serotonin*, *dopamine*, and *tyramine* (an intermediate in the conversion of tyrosine to norepinephrine).
- By **irreversibly** inhibiting the enzymes MAO-A and -B, MAOIs ↑ the number of neurotransmitters available in synapses.
- MAO-A preferentially deactivates serotonin and norepinephrine, and MAO-B preferentially deactivates phenethylamine; *both* types also act on dopamine and tyramine.
- MAOIs are not used as first-line agents because of the ↑ safety and tolerability of newer agents, notably SSRIs/SNRIs. However, MAOIs are used for certain types of **refractory depression** and in refractory anxiety disorders:
  - **Phenelzine (Nardil)**
  - **Tranylcypromine (Parnate)**
  - **Isocarboxazid (Marplan)**

Side Effects

- **Serotonin syndrome** occurs when **SSRIs** and **MAOIs** are taken together or if other drugs cause ↑ serotonin levels.
  - Initially characterized by lethargy, restlessness, confusion, flushing, diaphoresis, tremor, and myoclonic jerks.
  - May progress to hyperthermia, hypertonicity, rhabdomyolysis, renal failure, convulsions, coma, and death.
  - Wait at least 2 weeks before switching from SSRI to MAOI, and at least 5–6 weeks with fluoxetine.
- **Hypertensive crisis:** Risk when MAOIs are taken with tyramine-rich foods or sympathomimetics.
  - Foods with tyramine (red wine, cheese, chicken liver, fava beans, cured meats) cause a buildup of stored catecholamines.
  - In addition to a markedly elevated BP, it is also characterized by headache, sweating, nausea and vomiting, photophobia, autonomic instability, chest pain, arrhythmias, and death.
- Orthostatic hypotension (most common).
- Drowsiness.
- Weight gain.
- Sexual dysfunction.
- Dry mouth.
- Sleep dysfunction.
- Patients with pyridoxine deficiency can have numbness or paresthesias, so they should supplement with B_6.
- Liver toxicity, seizures, and edema (rare).
- *"Start low and go slow"* (low doses that are ↑ slowly).

Antidepressant Use in Other Disorders

- OCD: SSRIs (in high doses), TCAs (clomipramine)
- Panic disorder: SSRIs, TCAs, MAOIs
- Eating disorders: SSRIs (in high doses), TCAs
- Persistent depressive disorder (dysthymia): SSRIs, SNRIs (e.g., venlafaxine, duloxetine)
- Social anxiety disorder (social phobia): SSRIs, SNRIs, MAOIs
- GAD: SSRIs, SNRIs (venlafaxine), TCAs
- Posttraumatic stress disorder: SSRIs

WARDS TIP

Selegiline (Emsam transdermal patch) is a MAOI used to treat depression that does not require following the dietary restrictions when used in low dosages. However, decongestants, opiates (such as meperidine, fentanyl, and tramadol), and serotonergic drugs must still be avoided.

WARDS TIP

First step when suspecting serotonin syndrome: Discontinue the medication(s). Next, provide supportive care and benzodiazepines. The serotonin antagonist cyproheptadine can also be used.

KEY FACT

Wellbutrin (bupropion) can lower the seizure threshold, but it is *not* associated with the sexual side effects of other antidepressants.

KEY FACT

Dry mouth, urinary retention, constipation, and blurry vision are some of the side effects of TCAs, caused by the anticholinergic effects.

- Irritable bowel syndrome: SSRIs, TCAs
- Enuresis: TCAs (imipramine)
- Neuropathic pain: TCAs (amitriptyline and nortriptyline), SNRIs
- Chronic pain: SNRIs, TCAs
- Fibromyalgia: SNRIs
- Migraine headaches: TCAs (amitriptyline)
- Smoking cessation: Bupropion
- Premenstrual dysphoric disorder: SSRIs
- Insomnia: Mirtazapine, trazodone, TCAs (doxepin)

Antipsychotics

- Antipsychotics are used to treat psychotic disorders as well as psychotic symptoms associated with other psychiatric and medical illnesses.
  - *Typical* or *first-generation* antipsychotics, sometimes referred to as neuroleptics, are classified according to potency and treat psychosis by blocking dopamine (D2) receptors.
  - *Atypical* or *second-generation* antipsychotics block both dopamine (D2) and serotonin (2A) receptors.
- Most antipsychotics have a number of actions and receptor interactions in the brain that contribute to their varied efficacy and side-effect profiles.
- Both typical and atypical antipsychotics have similar efficacies in treating the presence of *positive psychotic symptoms*, such as hallucinations and delusions.
- Atypical antipsychotics were thought to be more effective at treating *negative symptoms* (such as flattened affect and social withdrawal), although this has not been consistently shown in the literature.
- Atypical antipsychotics have largely replaced typical antipsychotics in use due to their favorable side-effect profile. However, evidence for metabolic syndrome, including weight gain, and other side effects, as well as the significant cost of these medications, means that currently both classes are used as first-line treatments.
- The choice of which specific medication to prescribe should be made based on the patient's individual clinical presentation, past response (favorable and unfavorable), side-effect profile, and patient preference.

TYPICAL (FIRST-GENERATION) ANTIPSYCHOTICS

All typical antipsychotics have similar efficacy, but vary in potency.

Low-Potency, Typical Antipsychotics
- Lower affinity for dopamine receptors and therefore a higher dose is required. Remember, *potency* refers to the action on dopamine receptors, *not* the level of efficacy.
- Higher incidence of antiadrenergic, anticholinergic, and antihistaminic side effects compared to high-potency typical antipsychotics.
- Lower incidence of EPS and (possibly) neuroleptic malignant syndrome.
- More lethality in overdose due to QTc prolongation and the potential for heart block and ventricular tachycardia.
- Rare risk for agranulocytosis, and slightly higher seizure risk than high-potency antipsychotics.
  - **Chlorpromazine (Thorazine):**
    - Commonly causes orthostatic hypotension
    - Can cause blue-gray skin discoloration

WARDS TIP

Warning about atypical antipsychotics: Although they are used to treat the behavioral symptoms of dementia and delirium, studies show an ↑ risk of all-cause mortality and stroke when using these agents in the elderly.

- Can → photosensitivity
- Also used to treat nausea and vomiting, as well as intractable hiccups
  - **Thioridazine (Mellaril):** Associated with retinitis pigmentosa

Midpotency, Typical Antipsychotics
- Have midrange properties.
  - **Loxapine (Loxitane):**
    - Higher risk of seizures.
    - Metabolite is an antidepressant.
  - **Thiothixene (Navane):** Can cause ocular pigment changes
  - **Molindone (Moban)**
  - **Perphenazine (Trilafon)**

High-Potency, Typical Antipsychotics
- Greater affinity for dopamine receptors; therefore a relatively low dose is needed to achieve effect.
- Less sedation, orthostatic hypotension, and anticholinergic effects.
- Greater risk for extrapyramidal symptoms and (likely) TD.
  - **Haloperidol (Haldol):** Can be given PO/IM/IV. Decanoate (long acting) form available
  - **Fluphenazine (Prolixin):** Decanoate form available
  - **Trifluoperazine (Stelazine):** Approved for nonpsychotic anxiety
  - **Pimozide (Orap):** Associated with QTc prolongation and ventricular tachycardia

Side Effects

- The positive symptoms of schizophrenia are treated by action of the medications in the mesolimbic dopamine pathway. The mesolimbic pathway includes the nucleus accumbens, the fornix, the amygdala, and the hippocampus.
- The negative symptoms of schizophrenia are thought to occur due to (decreased) dopaminergic action in the mesocortical pathway.
- Extrapyramidal symptoms occur through blockade of the dopamine pathways in the nigrostriatum.
- ↑ prolactin is caused by dopamine blockade in the tuberoinfundibular area.
- **Antidopaminergic effects:**
  - EPS:
    - *Parkinsonism*—bradykinesia, masklike face, cogwheel rigidity, pill-rolling tremor.
    - *Akathisia*—subjective anxiety and restlessness, objective fidgetiness. Patients may report a sensation of inability to sit still. Best treated with B-blockers or benzodiazepines.
    - *Dystonia*—sustained painful contraction of muscles of neck (*torticollis*), tongue, eyes (*oculogyric crisis*). It can be life threatening if it involves the airway or diaphragm.
  - **Hyperprolactinemia**—→ ↓ libido, galactorrhea, gynecomastia, impotence, amenorrhea.
- **Anti-HAM effects:** Caused by actions on **H**istaminic, **A**drenergic, and **M**uscarinic receptors:
  - *Antihistaminic*—results in sedation, **weight gain**.
  - *Anti–α1 adrenergic*—results in orthostatic hypotension, cardiac abnormalities, and sexual dysfunction.
  - *Antimuscarinic*—anticholinergic effects, resulting in dry mouth, tachycardia, urinary retention, blurry vision, constipation, and precipitation of narrow-angle glaucoma.

- **Tardive dyskinesia:**
  - Choreoathetoid (writhing) movements of mouth and tongue (or other body parts) that may occur in patients who have used neuroleptics for >6 months.
  - Older age is a risk factor.
  - Women and patients with affective disorders *may* be at an increased risk.
  - Although 50% of cases will spontaneously remit (without further antipsychotic use), most cases are *permanent*.
  - Treatment involves discontinuation of current antipsychotic if clinically possible and changing to a medication with less potential to cause TD.
- Less common side effects include **neuroleptic malignant syndrome:**
  - Though rare, occurs more often in *young males early in treatment* with *high-potency typical antipsychotics*.
  - It is a **medical emergency** and has up to a 20% mortality rate if left untreated.
  - It is characterized by:
    - Fever (most common presenting symptom)
    - Autonomic instability (tachycardia, labile hypertension, diaphoresis)
    - Leukocytosis
    - Tremor
    - Elevated CPK
    - Rigidity (*lead pipe* rigidity is considered almost universal)
    - Excessive sweating (diaphoresis)
    - Delirium (mental status changes)
  - **Treatment** involves discontinuation of current medications and administration of supportive medical care (hydration, cooling, etc.).
  - Sodium dantrolene, bromocriptine, and amantadine may be used but have their own side effects and unclear efficacy.
  - This is *not* an allergic reaction.
  - Patient is not prevented from restarting the same neuroleptic at a later time, but will have an increased risk for another episode of neuroleptic malignant syndrome.
- Elevated liver enzymes, jaundice.
- **Ophthalmologic** problems (irreversible retinal pigmentation with high doses of thioridazine, deposits in lens and cornea with chlorpromazine).
- **Dermatologic** problems, including rashes and photosensitivity (blue-gray skin discoloration with chlorpromazine).
- **Seizures:** All antipsychotics lower the seizure threshold, although low-potency antipsychotics are more likely.

Ms. Brown is a 28-year-old, overweight woman who presents to your outpatient clinic following discharge from an inpatient psychiatry unit. Police found her in a local shopping mall, talking to herself and telling passersby that the devil had "stolen her soul." She appeared disheveled and scared. During the hospitalization, she was diagnosed with schizophrenia, and olanzapine was prescribed and titrated to 30 mg at bedtime for delusional thinking and disorganized behavior. She has since been living with her parents, and her hygiene and self-care have improved. Although Ms. Brown reports occasional auditory hallucinations telling her that her parents do not like her, she recognizes that the voices are not real and is not distressed by them. Ms. Brown has become involved in a vocational skills program and hopes to work at a local supermarket. However, during her last appointment with her primary care doctor, she was told she had an elevated fasting glucose of 115 and triglycerides of 180, and that she had gained 12 pounds in the past 3 months with a waist circumference of 36 inches. Her blood pressure was normal, but she reported a family history of diabetes and high blood pressure.

What is the next step?

Given her diagnosis of schizophrenia, and that Ms. Brown has had an adequate partial response to pharmacological treatment, she should continue to be treated with an antipsychotic. However, her recent laboratory results are suggestive of metabolic syndrome, and thus she is at an ↑ risk for cardiovascular disease. While this patient has responded well to olanzapine, this medication along with other atypical antipsychotics have been associated with ↑ weight gain and impaired glucose metabolism. It is unclear if Ms. Brown's laboratory test results were abnormal prior to starting olanzapine, are elevated secondary to treatment, or a combination of both. In treating Ms. Brown, first steps include recommending lifestyle modifications and close monitoring of her weight, blood sugar levels, lipids, and waist circumference, while collaborating closely with her primary care physician. If a change in her antipsychotic medication is warranted after weighing the risks and benefits of altering her treatment, other atypical antipsychotics such as ziprasidone or aripiprazole (less associated with weight gain), or typical antipsychotics might be considered; these medications would then be cross-tapered. When choosing medications, consideration must be given to a history of response, tolerability, side-effect profile, patient preference, and cost.

> **WARDS TIP**
>
> Onset of Antipsychotic side effects
> NMS: Any time (but usually early in treatment)
> Acute dystonia: Hours to days
> Parkinsonism/Akathisia: Days to weeks
> TD: Months to years
> The Abnormal Involuntary Movement Scale (AIMS) can be used to quantify and monitor for tardive dyskinesia.

ATYPICAL (SECOND-GENERATION) ANTIPSYCHOTICS

- Atypical antipsychotics block both dopamine and serotonin receptors and are associated with different side effects than typical antipsychotics.
- In particular, they are less likely to cause EPS, TD, or neuroleptic malignant syndrome.
- They *may* be more effective in treating **negative symptoms** of schizophrenia than typical antipsychotics.
- Atypical antipsychotics are also used to treat acute mania, bipolar disorder, and as adjunctive medications in unipolar depression.
- They are also used in treating borderline personality disorder, PTSD, and certain psychiatric disorders in childhood (e.g., tic disorders).
  - **Clozapine (Clozaril):**
    - Less likely to cause TD.
    - Only antipsychotic shown to be **more efficacious**; used in **treatment refractory schizophrenia**.
    - Associated with tachycardia and hypersalivation.
    - More anticholinergic side effects than other atypical or high-potency typical antipsychotics.
    - Small risk of **myocarditis**.
    - 1% incidence of **agranulocytosis**.
    - Clozapine must be stopped if the *absolute neutrophil count* drops below 1500/microliter.
    - 4% incidence of **seizures**.
    - Only antipsychotic shown to ↓ **the risk of suicide**.

> **WARDS TIP**
>
> Thirty percent of patients with treatment-resistant psychosis will respond to clozapine.

> **KEY FACT**
>
> Haldol has an increased risk of extrapyramidal side effects such as dystonia and tardive dyskinesia, but does not typically lead to agranulocytosis, which is associated with clozapine.

- **Risperidone (Risperdal):**
    - Can cause ↑ prolactin
    - Orthostatic hypotension and reflex tachycardia
    - Long-acting injectable form named Consta
- **Quetiapine (Seroquel):** Much less likely to cause EPS; common side effects include sedation and orthostatic hypotension.
- **Olanzapine (Zyprexa):** Common side effects include weight gain and sedation.
- **Ziprasidone (Geodon):** Less likely to cause significant weight gain, associated with QTc prolongation, and must be taken with food (50% reduction in absorption without a 300 calorie meal).
- **Aripiprazole (Abilify):**
    - Unique mechanism of partial D2 agonism
    - Can be more activating (akathisia) and less sedating
    - Less potential for weight gain
- Newer (more expensive) antipsychotics:
    - **Paliperidone (Invega):**
        - Metabolite of risperidone
        - Long-acting injectable form (Sustenna)
    - **Asenapine (Saphris)** Orally dissolving (sublingual) tablet
    - **Iloperidone (Fanapt)**
    - **Lurasidone (Latuda):** Must be taken with food; used in bipolar depression.

Side Effects

- **Metabolic syndrome.**
    - This must be monitored with baseline weight, waist circumference (measured at iliac crest), BP, fasting glucose, and fasting lipids.
    - **Weight gain.**
    - Hyperlipidemia.
    - Hyperglycemia—rarely, **diabetic ketoacidosis** has been reported.
- Some anti-HAM effects (antihistaminic, antiadrenergic, and antimuscarinic).
- Elevated liver function tests (LFTs)—monitor yearly for elevation in LFTs and ammonia.
- QTc prolongation.

Mood Stabilizers

- Mood stabilizers are used to treat **acute mania** and to help **prevent relapses** of manic episodes (maintenance treatment) in bipolar disorder and schizoaffective disorder. Less commonly, they may be used for:
    - Augmentation of antidepressants in patients with major depression refractory to monotherapy
    - Potentiation of antipsychotics in patients with schizophrenia or schizoaffective disorder
    - Treatment of aggression and impulsivity (e.g., neurocognitive disorders, intellectual disability, personality disorders, other medical conditions)
    - Enhancement of abstinence in treatment of alcoholism
- Mood stabilizers include lithium and anticonvulsants, most commonly valproic acid, lamotrigine, and carbamazepine.

LITHIUM

- Lithium is the drug of choice in acute mania and as prophylaxis for both manic and depressive episodes in bipolar and schizoaffective disorders.
- It is also used in cyclothymic disorder and unipolar depression.

WARDS TIP

Quetiapine, olanzapine, aripiprazole, risperidone, asenapine, and ziprasidone have FDA approval for treatment of mania.

WARDS TIP

Patients on clozapine must have weekly blood draws for the first 6 months to check WBC and absolute neutrophil counts because of the risk of agranulocytosis. With time, the frequency of blood draws ↓.

WARDS TIP

Antipsychotics may be used as adjuncts to mood stabilizers early in the course of a manic episode. Atypical antipsychotics are often prescribed as monotherapy in the acute or maintenance treatment of bipolar disorder.

KEY FACT

Lithium is the only mood stabilizer shown to ↓ suicidality.

- Lithium is metabolized by the kidney, so dosing adjustments may be necessary in patients with renal dysfunction.
- Prior to initiating, patients should have an ECG, basic chemistries, thyroid function tests, a complete blood count (CBC), and a pregnancy test.
- Onset of action takes 5–7 days.
- Blood levels correlate with clinical efficacy and should be checked after 5 days, and then every 2–3 days until therapeutic.
- The major drawback of lithium is its high incidence of side effects and very narrow therapeutic index:
  - Therapeutic range: 0.6–1.2 (Individual patients can have significant side effects even within this range.)
  - Toxic: >1.5
  - Potentially lethal: >2.0

Side Effects

- Toxic levels of lithium cause altered mental status, coarse tremors, convulsions, delirium, coma, and death.
- Clinicians need to regularly monitor blood levels of lithium, thyroid function (thyroid-stimulating hormone), and kidney function.
- Fine tremor.
- Nephrogenic diabetes insipidus.
- GI disturbance.
- Weight gain.
- Sedation.
- Thyroid enlargement, hypothyroidism.
- ECG changes.
- Benign leukocytosis.
- Lithium can cause **Ebstein's anomaly**, a cardiac defect in babies born to mothers taking lithium.

Anticonvulsants

CARBAMAZEPINE (TEGRETOL)

- Especially useful in treating mania with *mixed features* and *rapid-cycling* bipolar disorder; less effective for the depressed phase.
- Acts by blocking sodium channels and inhibiting action potentials.
- Onset of action is 5–7 days.
- CBC and LFTs must be obtained before initiating treatment and regularly monitored during treatment.

Side Effects

- The most common side effects are GI and CNS (e.g., drowsiness, ataxia, sedation, confusion).
- Possible skin rash **(Stevens–Johnson Syndrome).**
- Leukopenia, hyponatremia, aplastic anemia, thrombocytopenia, and agranulocytosis.
- Elevation of liver enzymes, causing hepatitis.
- **Teratogenic** effects when used during pregnancy (neural tube defects).
- Significant drug interactions with many medications metabolized by the cytochrome P450 pathway, including inducing its own metabolism through *autoinduction* (requiring increasing dosages).
- Toxicity: Confusion, stupor, motor restlessness, ataxia, tremor, nystagmus, twitching, and vomiting.

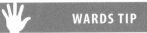

KEY FACT

When prescribing lithium, it is important to monitor lithium levels, creatinine, and thyroid function tests.

WARDS TIP

Blood levels are useful for lithium, valproic acid, carbamazapine, and clozapine.

WARDS TIP

Be careful of prescribing ibuprofen or other NSAIDs to a patient on lithium.

WARDS TIP

Factors that increase Li+ levels:
- NSAIDs
- Aspirin (+/−)
- Thiazide diuretics
- Dehydration
- Salt deprivation
- Sweating (salt loss)
- Impaired renal function

WARDS TIP

The side effect of leukocytosis can be advantageous when combined with other medications that ↓ WBC count (e.g., clozapine).

VALPROIC ACID (DEPAKOTE AND DEPAKENE)

- Useful in treating acute mania, mania with mixed features, and rapid cycling.
- Multiple mechanisms of action: blocks sodium channels and increases GABA concentrations in the brain.
- Monitoring of LFTs and CBC is necessary.
- Drug levels should be checked after 4–5 days. Therapeutic range is 50–150 µg/mL.
- Contraindicated in pregnancy so care should be given in women of child-bearing age (neural tube defects).

Lamotrigine (Lamictal)
- Efficacy for **bipolar depression,** though little efficacy for acute mania or prevention of mania.
- Believed to work on sodium channels that modulate glutamate and aspartate.
- Most common side effects are dizziness, sedation, headaches, and ataxia.
- Most serious side effect is **Stevens-Johnson syndrome** (life-threatening rash involving skin and mucous membranes) in 0.1%. This is most likely in the first 2–8 weeks, but is minimized by starting with low doses and increasing *slowly*.
- Valproate will ↑ lamotrigine levels, and lamotrigine will ↓ valproate levels.

Oxcarbazepine (Trileptal)
- As effective in mood disorders as carbamazepine, but better tolerated
- Less risk of rash and hepatic toxicity
- Monitor sodium levels for hyponatremia

Gabapentin (Neurontin)
- Often used adjunctively to help with anxiety, sleep, neuropathic pain
- Little efficacy in bipolar disorder

Pregabalin (Lyrica)
- Used in GAD (second-line) and fibromyalgia
- Little efficacy in bipolar disorder

Tiagabine (Gabitril): Questionable benefit in treating anxiety
Topiramate (Topamax)
- May be helpful with impulse control disorders
- Beneficial side effect is **weight loss**
- Can cause hypochloremic, metabolic acidosis, as well as kidney stones
- The most limiting side effect is **cognitive slowing**

Side Effects

- GI symptoms
- Weight gain
- Sedation
- Alopecia
- Pancreatitis
- **Hepatotoxicity** or benign aminotransferase elevations
- ↑ ammonia
- Thrombocytopenia
- **Teratogenic** effects during pregnancy (neural tube defects)

Anxiolytics/Hypnotics

- Include benzodiazepines (BDZs), barbiturates, and buspirone.
- BDZs are the most widely prescribed psychotropic medications.

WARDS TIP

In chronic alcoholics or liver disease, use benzodiazepines that are not metabolized by the liver. There are a LOT of them:
Lorazepam
Oxazepam
Temazepam

- Common indications for anxiolytics/hypnotics include:
  - Anxiety disorders
  - Muscle spasm
  - Seizures
  - Sleep disorders
  - Alcohol withdrawal
  - Anesthesia induction

BENZODIAZEPINES

- BDZs work by potentiating the effects of gamma-aminobutyric acid (GABA).
- They reduce anxiety and can be used to treat akathisia.
- Many patients become physically dependent on these medications and require increasing amounts for the same clinical effect (i.e., tolerance).
- Potential for abuse.
- Choice of BDZ is based on time to onset of action, duration of action, and method of metabolism.
- Relatively safer in overdose than barbiturates.
- **Long Acting (Half-life: >20 Hours)**
- **Diazepam (Valium):**
  - Rapid onset
  - Used during detoxification from alcohol or sedative-hypnotic-anxiolytics, and for seizures
  - Effective for muscle spasm
  - Less commonly prescribed to treat anxiety because of euphoria
- **Clonazepam (Klonopin):**
  - Treatment of anxiety, including panic attacks
  - Avoid with renal dysfunction; longer half-life allows for once or twice daily dosing
- **Intermediate Acting (Half-life: 6–20 Hours)**
- **Alprazolam (Xanax):**
  - Treatment of anxiety, including panic attacks
  - Shorter onset of action → euphoria, high abuse potential
- **Lorazepam (Ativan):**
  - Treatment of panic attacks, alcohol and sedative-hypnotic-anxiolytic detoxification, agitation
  - Not metabolized by liver
- **Oxazepam (Serax):**
  - Alcohol and sedative-hypnotic-anxiolytic detoxification
  - Not metabolized by liver
- **Temazepam (Restoril):**
  - Because of dependence, decreasingly used for treatment of insomnia
  - Not metabolized by liver
- **Short Acting (Half-life: <6 Hours)**
- **Triazolam (Halcion):**
  - Treatment of insomnia
  - Risk of anterograde amnesia and sleep-related activities (e.g., eating, driving)
- **Midazolam (Versed):**
  - **Very short half-life**
  - Primarily used in medical and surgical settings

Side Effects

- Drowsiness
- Impairment of intellectual function
- Reduced motor coordination (careful in elderly)

WARDS TIP

BDZs can be lethal when mixed with alcohol. Respiratory depression may cause death.

WARDS TIP

For benzodiazepine overdose, flumazenil is used to reverse the effects. However, be careful not to induce withdrawal too quickly—this can be life threatening.

- Anterograde amnesia
- Withdrawal can be life threatening and cause seizures
- Toxicity: Respiratory depression in overdose, especially when combined with alcohol

NON-BDZ HYPNOTICS

- **Zolpidem (Ambien)/zaleplon (Sonata)/eszopiclone (Lunesta):**
  - Work by selective receptor binding to the omega-1 receptor on the GABA-A receptor, which is responsible for sedation.
  - Should be used for short-term treatment of insomnia.
  - Compared to BDZs, less tolerance/dependence occurs with prolonged use (but still can occur).
  - Zaleplon has a shorter half-life than zolpidem, which has a shorter half-life than eszopiclone.
  - Reports of anterograde amnesia, hallucinations, parasomnias (sleep-walking), and GI side effects may limit their tolerability.
- **Diphenhydramine (Benadryl):**
  - An antihistamine with moderate anticholinergic effects.
  - Side effects include sedation, dry mouth, constipation, urinary retention, and blurry vision.
- **Ramelteon (Rozerem):**
  - Selective melatonin MT_1 and MT_2 agonist
  - No tolerance or dependence

NON-BDZ ANXIOLYTICS

- **Buspirone (BuSpar):**
  - Partial agonist at 5HT-1A receptor.
  - Slower onset of action than BDZs (takes 1–2 weeks for effect).
  - Not considered as effective as other options, and so it is often used in combination with another agent (e.g., an SSRI) for the treatment of generalized anxiety disorder.
  - Does not potentiate the CNS depression of alcohol (useful in alcoholics), and has a low potential for abuse/addiction.
- **Hydroxyzine (Atarax):**
  - An antihistamine.
  - Side effects include sedation, dry mouth, constipation, urinary retention, and blurry vision.
  - Useful for patients who want quick-acting, short-term medication, but who cannot take BDZs for various reasons.
- **Barbiturates** (e.g., **butalbitol, phenobarbital, amobarbitol, pentobarbital**): Rarely used because of the lethality of overdose, potential for abuse, and side-effect profile.
- **Propranolol:**
  - Beta-blocker.
  - Useful in treating the autonomic effects of panic attacks or social phobia (i.e., performance anxiety), such as palpitations, sweating, and tachycardia.
  - It can also be used to treat akathisia (side effect of antipsychotics).

Psychostimulants

Used in ADHD and in treatment refractory depression.
- **Dextroamphetamine and amphetamines (Dexedrine, Adderall):**
  - Dextroamphetamine is the d-isomer of amphetamine.

- Schedule II due to high potential for **abuse/diversion.**
- Monitor BP, and watch for weight loss, insomnia, exacerbation of tics, decreased seizure threshold
- **Methylphenidate (Ritalin, Concerta):**
  - CNS stimulant, similar to amphetamine.
  - Schedule II.
  - Watch for leukopenia or anemia.
  - Monitor BP and CBC with differential, and watch for weight loss, insomnia, exacerbation of tics, decreased seizure threshold.
- **Atomoxetine (Strattera):**
  - Inhibits presynaptic norepinephrine reuptake, resulting in increased synaptic norepinephrine and dopamine.
  - Less appetite suppression and insomnia.
  - Not classified as a controlled substance.
  - Less abuse potential than dextroamphetamine/methylphenidate but less effective.
  - Rare liver toxicity, and possible ↑ SI in children/adolescents.
- **Modafinil (Provigil):** Used in narcolepsy, not ADHD

Cognitive Enhancers

Used in major neurocognitive disorders (dementias).

ACETYLCHOLINESTERASE INHIBITORS

- **Donepezil (Aricept):**
  - Once-daily dosing
  - Some GI side effects
  - Used in mild to moderate neurocognitive disorders (dementias)
- **Galantamine (Razadyne):**
  - Twice-daily dosing
  - GI side effects
  - Used in mild to moderate neurocognitive disorders (dementias)
- **Rivastigmine (Exelon):**
  - Twice-daily dosing
  - Has daily patch form, with fewer side effects
  - Used in mild to moderate neurocognitive disorders (dementias)

> **KEY FACT**
>
> Alzheimer's medications, such as donepezil and rivastigmine, work by reversible inhibition of acetylcholine esterase.

NMDA (GLUTAMATE) RECEPTOR ANTAGONIST

- **Memantine (Namenda):**
  - Used in moderate to severe neurocognitive disorders (dementia)
  - Fewer side effects than cholinesterase inhibitors
  - Should be used with acetylcholinesterase inhibitor

Summary of Medications That May Cause Psychiatric Symptoms

PSYCHOSIS

Sympathomimetics, analgesics, antibiotics (e.g., isoniazid, antimalarials), anticholinergics, anticonvulsants, antihistamines, corticosteroids, antiparkinsonian agents.

AGITATION/CONFUSION/DELIRIUM

Antipsychotics, **anticholinergics**, **antihistamines**, antidepressants, antiarrhythmics, antineoplastics, corticosteroids, nonsteroidal anti-inflammatories (NSAIDs), antiasthmatics, antibiotics, antihypertensives, antiparkinsonian agents, thyroid hormones.

DEPRESSION

Antihypertensives, antiparkinsonian agents, **corticosteroids**, calcium channel blockers, NSAIDs, antibiotics, peptic ulcer drugs.

ANXIETY

Sympathomimetics, antiasthmatics, antiparkinsonian agents, hypoglycemic agents, NSAIDs, thyroid hormones.

SEDATION/POOR CONCENTRATION

Antianxiety agents/hypnotics, anticholinergics, antibiotics, antihistamines.

SELECTED MEDICATIONS

- **Procainamide, quinidine:** Confusion, delirium
- **Albuterol:** Anxiety, confusion
- **Isoniazid:** Psychosis
- **Tetracycline:** Depression
- **Nifedipine, verapamil:** Depression
- **Cimetidine:** Depression, confusion, psychosis
- **Steroids:** Aggressiveness/agitation, mania, depression, anxiety, psychosis

Other Treatments

ELECTROCONVULSIVE THERAPY (ECT)

Patients are often premedicated with atropine, and then given general anesthesia (typically with methohexital) and muscle relaxants (e.g., succinylcholine). A generalized tonic-clonic seizure is then induced using unilateral or bilateral electrodes. While the mechanism of action of ECT is not fully known, there are likely anticonvulsant effects, as well as brain perfusion and connectivity changes involved. ECT is **the most effective** treatment for major depressive disorder, especially with psychotic features, as well as for acute mania and catatonia. It is often used in patients who cannot tolerate medications or who have failed other treatments. ECT is discontinued after symptomatic improvement, typically a course of 8–12 sessions given three times weekly. Monthly *maintenance ECT* is often used to prevent relapse of symptoms. The most common side effects are muscle soreness, headaches, amnesia, and confusion. Bilateral electrode placement is more efficacious, but ↑ memory impairment and confusion.

DEEP BRAIN STIMULATION (DBS)

DBS is a surgical treatment involving the implantation of a medical device that sends electrical impulses to specific parts of the brain. DBS in select brain regions has provided benefits for Parkinson's disease and disabling dystonia, as well as for chronic pain and tremors. Its underlying principles and mechanisms are still not clear. DBS directly changes brain activity in a controlled manner and its effects are reversible (unlike those of lesioning techniques). DBS has been used to treat various affective disorders, including major depression. While DBS has proven helpful for some patients, there is potential for serious complications and side effects.

REPETITIVE TRANSCRANIAL MAGNETIC STIMULATION (rTMS)

rTMS is a noninvasive method to excite neurons in the brain. Weak electric currents are induced in the tissue by rapidly changing magnetic fields, a process called electromagnetic induction. In this way, brain activity can be triggered with minimal discomfort. rTMS can produce longer-lasting changes than nonrepetitive stimulation. Numerous small-scale studies have demonstrated efficacy in the treatment of major depression; however, studies show less efficacy than for ECT, and the price of treatment is high. Side effects include seizures (rare), as well as headache and scalp pain.

LIGHT THERAPY

Light therapy, or phototherapy, consists of exposure to daylight or to specific wavelengths of light using lasers, light-emitting diodes, fluorescent lamps, dichroic lamps or very bright, full-spectrum light, for a prescribed amount of time and, in some cases, at a specific time of day. Light therapy is used to treat major depression with a seasonal pattern (**seasonal affective disorder**), with some support for its use with nonseasonal psychiatric disorders.

CHAPTER 19

FORENSIC PSYCHIATRY

Standard of Care and Malpractice	210	Disability	212
Confidentiality	210	Competence to Stand Trail	212
Decision Making	211	Not Guilty by Reason of Insanity (NGRI)	213
EMANCIPATED MINORS	211	Risk Assessment	213
DECISIONAL CAPACITY	211	Other Areas of Forensic Psychiatry	213
GUARDIANS AND CONSERVATORS	211	CHILD AND FAMILY LAW	214
Admission to a Psychiatric Hospital	212	CORRECTIONAL PSYCHIATRY	214

Forensic psychiatry is a medical subspecialty that includes the areas in which psychiatry is applied to legal issues. Forensic psychiatrists often conduct evaluations requested by the court or attorneys.

While some forensic psychiatrists specialize exclusively in legal issues, almost all psychiatrists have to work within one of the many spheres where the mental health and legal system overlap. These areas include the following:

- Risk assessment
- Criminal responsibility
- Competence/decisional capacity
- Child custody and visitation
- Psychic injury
- Mental disability
- Malpractice
- Involuntary treatment
- Correctional psychiatry

Legal issues are considered **criminal** in nature if someone is being charged with a crime. **Civil** cases involve other kinds of rights and may result in monetary awards. The specific laws pertaining to the various topics discussed in this chapter often vary by state.

Standard of Care and Malpractice

- The **standard of care** in psychiatry is generally defined as the skill level and knowledge base of the average, prudent psychiatrist in a given community.
- **Negligence** is practicing below the standard of care.
- **Malpractice** is the act of being negligent as a doctor.
- The following four conditions must be proven by a preponderance of the evidence to sustain a claim of malpractice:
  1. The physician had a duty of care (psychiatrist–patient relationship).
  2. The physician breached his or her duty by practice that did not meet the standard of care (negligence).
  3. The patient was harmed.
  4. The harm was directly caused by the physician's negligence.
- If a malpractice case is successful, the patient can receive **compensatory damages** (reimbursement for medical expenses, lost salary, or physical suffering) and **punitive damages** (money awarded to "punish" the doctor).

Confidentiality

All information regarding a doctor–patient relationship should be held confidential, except when otherwise exempted by statute, such as:

- When sharing relevant information with other staff members who are also treating the patient.
- If subpoenaed—physician must supply all requested information.
- If child abuse is suspected—obligated to report to the proper authorities.
- If a patient is suicidal—physician may need to admit the patient, with or without the patient's consent, and share information with the hospital staff.

WARDS TIP

A wrong prediction or a bad outcome is not necessarily proof of bad doctoring (malpractice).

KEY FACT

4 Ds of malpractice: Deviation (neglect) from Duty that was the Direct cause of Damage

KEY FACT

The obligation of a physician to report patients who are potentially dangerous to others is called the *Tarasoff duty* or *duty to warn*, based on a landmark legal case.

Decision Making

- Process by which patients knowingly and voluntarily agree to a treatment or procedure.
- In order to make informed decisions, patients must know the purpose of the treatment, alternative treatments, and the potential risks and benefits of undergoing and of refusing the treatment.
- The patient should have the opportunity to ask questions.
- Situations that do not require informed consent:
    - Lifesaving medical emergency
    - Prevention of suicidal or homicidal behavior
    - Unemancipated minors

EMANCIPATED MINORS

- Considered competent to give consent for all medical care without parental input or consent
- Minors are considered emancipated if they are:
    - Self-supporting
    - In the military
    - Married
    - Have children **or pregnant**

DECISIONAL CAPACITY

Competence and *capacity* are terms that refer to a patient's ability to make informed treatment decisions.

- *Capacity* is a clinical term and may be assessed by physicians.
- *Competence* is a legal term and can be decided only by a judge.
- Decisional capacity is *task specific* and can fluctuate over time.
- In order for a patient to have decisional capacity, he or she must be able to:
    - Understand the relevant information regarding treatment (purpose, risks, benefits).
    - Appreciate the appropriate weight and impact of the decision.
    - Logically manipulate the information to make a decision.
    - Communicate a choice or preference.
- Criteria for determining capacity may be more stringent if the consequences of a patient's decision are very serious.
- If a patient is determined not to have decisional capacity, the decision is typically made by a surrogate decision maker, usually a power of attorney, spouse, or close family member.

GUARDIANS AND CONSERVATORS

- May be appointed by a judge to make treatment decisions for incompetent patients.
- Should make decisions by substituted judgment (what the patient would most likely have expressed were the patient competent).

KEY FACT

- Elements of informed consent (4 Rs):
- Reason for treatment
- Risks and benefits
- Reasonable alternatives
- Refused treatment consequences

KEY FACT

Emancipated minors do not need parental consent to make medical decisions.

Admission to a Psychiatric Hospital

The two main categories of admission to a psychiatric hospital are voluntary and involuntary.

- **Voluntary:**
  - Patient requests or agrees to be admitted to the psychiatric ward.
  - Voluntary patients may not have the right to be discharged immediately upon request.
  - Patient must have capacity and be competent to be admitted as a voluntary patient to an inpatient facility.
- **Involuntary:**
  - Patient must be found to be harmful to self or others or unable to provide for his/her basic needs.
  - Involuntary patients have legal rights to a trial to challenge their hospitalization.
  - Involuntary patients do not automatically lose the right to refuse treatment, including the involuntary administration of medication.
  - Involuntary commitment is supported by legal principles of **police power** (protecting citizens from each other) and **parens patriae** (protecting citizens who can't care for themselves).

> **KEY FACT**
>
> Doctors are required to report child abuse, but lawyers are not.

> **WARDS TIP**
>
> If a child presents to the emergency department with various bruises, suspicious injuries in various stages of healing, and numerous prior emergency room visits, your next step would most likely be to contact appropriate authorities.

Disability

- **Mental impairment:** Any mental or psychological disorder
- **Mental disability:** Alteration of an individual's capacity to meet personal, social, or occupational demands due to a mental impairment
- To assess whether an impairment is also a disability, consider four categories:
  - Activities of daily living
  - Social functioning
  - Concentration, persistence, and pace
  - Deterioration or decomposition in work settings

Competence to Stand Trail

- *Competence* is a legal term for the capacity to understand, rationally manipulate, and apply information to make a reasoned decision on a specific issue. This definition varies by state.
- The 6th and 14th Amendments to the Constitution are the basis for the law that someone cannot be tried if they are not mentally competent to stand trial.
- This was established by the legal case *Dusky v. United States* in 1960.
- If a defendant has significant mental health problems or behaves irrationally in court, his competency to stand trial should be considered.
- Competence may change over time.
- To stand trial, a defendant must:
  - Understand the charges against him or her.
  - Be familiar with the courtroom personnel.
  - Have the ability to work with an attorney and participate in his or her trial.
  - Understand possible consequences.

> **KEY FACT**
>
> 6th Amendment: Right to counsel, a speedy trial, and to confront witnesses

> **KEY FACT**
>
> 14th Amendment: Right to due process of law

> **KEY FACT**
>
> The fact that someone is mentally ill doesn't mean they aren't competent to stand trial.

Not Guilty by Reason of Insanity (NGRI)

- Conviction of a crime requires both an "evil deed" (*actus reus*) and "evil intent" (*mens rea*).
- **Insanity** is a legal term, and its definition varies by state (see Table 19-1).
- If someone is declared legally insane, they are not criminally responsible for their act.
- Some states have a ruling of Guilty but Mentally Ill (GBMI) instead of NGRI, or no criminal insanity defense at all.
- NGRI is used in <1% of criminal cases.
- It is successful in 26% of cases that continue to use it throughout the trial.
- Those found NGRI often spend the same amount of time (or more) as involuntary psychiatric patients than they would have spent in prison if they were found guilty.

Risk Assessment

- Mental disorders are neither necessary, nor sufficient causes of violence.
    - The major risk factors of violence are a history of violence, being young, male, and of lower socioeconomic status.
    - Substance use is a major determinant of violence, whether it occurs in the context of a mental illness or not.
- **Predicting dangerousness:**
    - Short-term easier than long-term
    - High false positives because of low base rates (most people are not violent)

Other Areas of Forensic Psychiatry

- *Frye v. United States* (1923): Evidence must be generally accepted by the appropriate scientific community.
- *Daubert v. Merrell Dow Pharmaceuticals* (1993): Judge decides if evidence is based on relevant and reliable science.

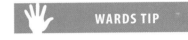
WARDS TIP

After John Hinckley received NGRI for an assassination attempt on President Reagan, there was public outcry against lenient NGRI standards, contributing to the Insanity Defense Reform Act of 1984.

WARDS TIP

The most important factor in assessing a patient's risk of violence is the individual's history of violence.

WARDS TIP

The contribution of people with mental illness to overall rates of violence is small. People with mental illness are more likely to be the *victims* of violence than the perpetrators.

TABLE 19-1.   Insanity Defense Standards

STANDARD	DEFINITION
M'Naghten	- Person did not understand what he/she was doing *or* its wrongfulness. - Most stringent test.
American Law Institute (ALI) Model Penal Code	Person could neither appreciate the criminality of his/her conduct *nor* conform his conduct to the requirements of the law.
Irresistible Impulse	Person could not appreciate right from wrong *or* could not control actions.
Durham	- The person's criminal act has resulted from mental illness. - Most lenient test and is rarely used.

- Malingering: Feigning or exaggerating symptoms for "secondary gain," including:
    - Financial gain (injury law suit)
    - Avoiding school, work, or other responsibilities
    - Obtaining medications of abuse (opioids, benzodiazepines)
    - Avoiding legal consequences
- Signs for detecting malingering:
    - Atypical presentation
    - "Textbook" description of the illness
    - History of working in the medical field
    - Symptoms that are present only when the patient knows he/she is being observed
    - History of substance use or antisocial personality disorder

CHILD AND FAMILY LAW

Evaluations for which a child forensic psychiatrist may be needed, include:

- Child custody
- Termination of parental rights
- Child abuse or neglect

CORRECTIONAL PSYCHIATRY

- With the closing of state psychiatric hospitals (i.e., deinstutionalization), many persons with mental illness have moved to correctional institutions.
- Psychiatrists who practice in jails and prisons must balance treating the inmates as their patients and maintaining safety in the institution.
- Issues of **confidentiality** and **violence** are key.

A 74-year-old African-American male with insulin-dependent diabetes mellitus and severe major depressive disorder was admitted to the intensive care unit for treatment of diabetic ketoacidosis. The internal medicine team calls your psychiatry consult-liaison service to evaluate the patient for depression and provide treatment recommendations.

When you meet the patient, he is disoriented, confused, and has a waxing and waning level of consciousness. His mini-mental state exam (MMSE) score is 18/30. You identify that the patient is likely delirious, and you are unable to obtain any useful historical information. After interviewing the patient's daughter by phone, you learn that the patient's wife passed away 2 years ago, and in the past he had told family members that he can no longer live without her. One year ago, his daughter found him in the garage taping a hose to his car's exhaust pipe. She said that he broke down crying and admitted that he was going to kill himself by carbon monoxide poisoning. His daughter has been very concerned because he refuses to check his glucose or take his insulin as recommended. She stated, "I think he was trying to kill himself by not taking care of his diabetes."

He is followed daily by your consult-liaison team, and his mental state improves each day. His MMSE score improves to 28/30. On hospital day 5, the internal medicine team informs you that he has developed wet gangrene in his right lower extremity and will need to have a below-knee amputation as soon as possible. The team asks you to assess the patient's capacity to make medical decisions, because he is adamantly refusing to consent to this procedure.

You meet with the patient to discuss his medical situation. He is alert, lucid, and fully oriented. His affect is euthymic and appropriate. He states, "My doctor told me that I had an ulcer on my foot from poorly controlled diabetes that has become severely infected. I was told that I need to have my right leg amputated very soon or else I could die from the infection." He maintains that he is not interested in the surgical procedure that has been recommended. He adds, "My daughter is begging me to have the surgery, but I'm already old and I don't want to have to use a prosthetic leg or a wheelchair. I do not think life would be worth living if I had this amputation." He denies suicidal thoughts and intent.

Does this patient with history of severe major depressive disorder demonstrate the capacity to refuse a potentially life-saving procedure?

Yes, he demonstrates the capacity to refuse the recommended amputation. Legal standards for decision-making capacity to consent or refuse medical treatment involve the following: the ability to communicate a choice, to understand the relevant information, to appreciate the medical consequences of the situation, and to reason about treatment choices. In this case, the patient demonstrated the ability to discuss all of these topics. Although he was cognitively impaired on admission, his delirium eventually cleared.

However, the case is complicated by the fact that the patient may be currently suffering from major depression; this should be further assessed. While a history of or current major depression does not preclude having decisional capacity, the patient should be evaluated carefully to ensure that his refusal of treatment does not stem from intent to commit suicide. If it does, then his suicidal intent would be interfering with his ability to reason. Optimally, the consult-liaison team may recommend treating the depression and readdressing the surgical procedure when his depression is in remission, but this may take many weeks and failure to amputate the limb in a timely manner could result in death. Since the patient demonstrates decision-making capacity and does not appear to be suicidal at this time, the medical team must respect the patient's wishes and treat the condition without surgery.

NOTES

INDEX

4 Ds of malpractice, 210
4 Ps (HPI), 13
5 A's of schizophrenia, 24
5 W's of NPH, 110

A

Abilify (aripiprazole), 197, 200
Acamprosate (Campral), 85
Acetylcholinesterase inhibitors, 205
Acting out, 182
Acute confusional state, 99
Acute dystonia, 9, 190
Acute insomnia, 160
Acute organic brain syndrome, 99
Acute stress disorder, 59
Acute toxic psychosis, 99
AD. *See* Alzheimer's disease (AD)
Adderall, 204–205
Addictive disorders. *See* Substance-related and
    addictive disorders
ADHD. *See* Attention deficit/hyperactivity
    disorder (ADHD)
Adjustment disorder, 60–61
Admission to psychiatric hospital, 212
Advanced sleep phase disorder, 166
Affect, 14–15
Affective disorders, 34. *See also* Mood disorders
AFRAID, 74
Agoraphobia, 51
Akathisia, 26, 190, 197
Akinesia, 13
Albuterol, 206
Alcohol (EtOH), 7, 48, 81–86
    alcohol use disorder, 85–86
    AST:ALT ratio, 85
    AUDIT-C, 86
    DTs, 83
    interactions with other medications, 118
    intoxication, 82
    Korsakoff syndrome, 86
    testing for substance use, 81
    Wernicke's encephalopathy, 86
    withdrawal, 83–84

Alcohol dehydrogenase, 82
Alcohol intoxication, 82
Alcohol use disorder, 85–86
Alcohol withdrawal symptoms, 83
Alcohol withdrawal syndrome, 83
Alcoholic hallucinosis, 16
Aldehyde dehydrogenase, 82
Alpha2-adrenergic receptor antagonists, 193
Alprazolam (Xanax), 203
Alprostadil, 175
Altruism, 181
Alzheimer's disease (AD), 104–105
Ambien (zolpidem), 89, 161, 204
Amitriptyline (Elavil), 161, 194
Amobarbital, 204
Amok, 31
Amoxapine (Asendin), 194
Amphetamines, 8, 48, 81, 87–88, 204–205
Anafranil (clomipramine), 194
Analytically oriented (psychodynamic)
    psychotherapy, 175
Angel dust, 88. *See also* Phencyclidine (PCP)
Anhedonia, 36
Anorexia nervosa, 153–154
Antabuse (disulfiram), 85
Anti-Ham effects, 197
Anticholinergic medications, 190
Anticonvulsants, 201–202
Antidepressants, 37–38, 191–196
    alpha2-adrenergic receptor antagonists, 193
    heterocyclic, 193–194
    norepinephrine-dopamine reuptake
        inhibitors, 193
    other disorders, 195–196
    serotonin receptor antagonists and agonists,
        193
    SNRIs, 192–193
    SSRIs, 191–192
    tetracyclic, 194
    tricyclic, 194
Antidopaminergic effects, 197
Antipsychotics, 27–29, 196–200
Antisocial personality disorder, 68, 69–70
Anxiety, 48

Anxiety disorders, 48–55
    agoraphobia, 51
    generalized anxiety disorder (GAD), 54–55
    medical conditions causing anxiety, 49
    medications/substances causing anxiety, 48
    pain attack, 49–50
    panic disorder, 50
    pharmacotherapy, 49
    psychotherapy, 49
    selective mutism, 52–53
    separation anxiety disorder, 53
    signs/symptoms of anxiety, 48
    social anxiety disorder, 51–52
    social phobia, 51–52
    specific phobias, 51–52
Anxiolytics, 48
Anxiolytics/hypnotics, 202–204
Apathetic thyrotoxicosis, 103
Aricept (donepezil), 105, 205
Aripiprazole (Abilify), 197, 200
Arson, 148
ASD. See Autism spectrum disorder (ASD)
Asenapine (Saphris), 200
Asendin (amoxapine), 194
AST:ALT ratio, 85
Atarax (hydroxyzine), 204
Ativan (lorazepam), 203
Atomoxetine (Strattera), 205
Attempted suicide, 83
Attention deficit/hyperactivity disorder (ADHD),
    125–126
Atypical antipsychotics, 28, 199–200
AUDIT-C, 86
Auditory hallucination, 22
Autism spectrum disorder (ASD), 126–127
Automatisms, 13
Aventyl (nortriptyline), 194
Aversion therapy, 184
Avoidant personality disorder, 73–74

B
Banana bag, 84
Barbiturate withdrawal, 89
Barbiturates, 7, 89
    CYP450 inducer, 190
    rarely used, 204
    testing for substance abuse, 81
    withdrawal, 89

BDZs. See Benzodiazepines (BDZs)
Bed-wetting, 130–131
Behavioral disinhibition, 118
Behavioral therapy, 184
Benadryl (diphenhydramine), 204
Benzodiazepine overdose, 203
Benzodiazepines (BDZs), 7, 89, 203–204
    anxiety, 49
    delirium, 102
    insomnia disorder, 161
    overdose, 203
    PTSD, 60
    side effects, 203–204
    testing for substance use, 81
Bereavement, 40, 117
Bereavement-associated depression, 117
Beta-blockers, 49
Binge eating, 155
Binge-eating disorder, 156–157
Binge-eating/purging-type anorexia, 153
Biofeedback, 184
Bipolar disorders, 40–42
Bipolar I disorder, 40–41
Bipolar II disorder, 41–42
Bizarre delusion, 22
Blood-injury-injection phobia, 52
Body dysmorphic disorder, 56
Borderline personality disorder (BPD), 68,
    70–71
BPD. See Borderline personality disorder (BPD)
Bradykinesia, 13, 190
Brain fag, 31
Breathing-related disorders, 160
Brief dynamic psychotherapy, 183
Brief psychotic disorder, 30
Bulimia nervosa, 155–156
Bullet presentation, 3–4
Buprenorphine, 91
Bupropion (Wellbutrin, Zyban), 94, 156,
    193, 195
Buspirone (BuSpar), 49, 204
Butalbital, 204

C
Caffeine, 8, 48, 93–94
Caffeine withdrawal symptoms, 94
CAM. See Confusion assessment method (CAM)
Campral (acamprosate), 85

Cannabis, 8, 48. *See also* Marijuana
Capacity, 211
CAPRI, 64
Carbamazepine (Tegretol), 190, 201
Carbidopa-levodopa, 109
Catatonia, 39, 42
Catatonic catalepsy, 165
CBT. *See* Cognitive-behavioral therapy (CBT)
Celexa (citalopram), 192
Central sleep apnea, 163
Chantix (varenicline), 94
CHASES, 42
Cheyne-Stokes breathing, 163
Child abuse, 131–132
Child and family law, 214
Child neglect, 132
Childhood-onset fluency disorder, 124
Children. *See* Pediatric psychiatry
Chlorpromazine (Thorazine), 196–197
Cholinesterase inhibitors, 105, 107, 109
Chronic insomnia, 160
Chronic motor or vocal tic disorder, 129
Cigarette smoking, 94. *See also* Nicotine
Cimetidine, 206
Circadian rhythm sleep wake disorders, 165–166
Circumstantiality, 15
Citalopram (Celexa), 192
Civil law, 210. *See also* Forensic psychiatry
CJD. *See* Creutzfeldt-Jakob disease (CJD)
Clang associations, 15
Classical conditioning, 184
Clerkship (shelf) examination, 4
Clomipramine (Anafranil), 194
Clonazepam (Klonopin), 107
Closed-ended questions, 12
Clozaril (clozapine), 24, 107, 109, 198, 199
Cluster A personality disorders, 64, 65–68
Cluster B personality disorders, 64, 68–73
Cluster C personality disorders, 64, 73–76
Cocaine, 8, 48, 81, 87
Cocaine use disorder, 87
Cognitive-behavioral therapy (CBT), 49, 185
  insomnia, 161
  sexual dysfunctions, 175
Cognitive distortions, 185
Cognitive enhancers, 205
Cognitive processing therapy, 60
Cognitive therapy, 185
Collaborative couples therapy, 187

Command hallucination, 22
Communication disorders, 124
Compensatory damages, 210
Competence, 211
Competence to stand trial, 212
Concerta. *See* Ritalin (methylphenidate)
Concurrent couples therapy, 187
Conditioning, 184
CONDUCT, 70
Conduct disorder, 129–130
Confabulations, 84
Confidentiality, 210
Confusion assessment method (CAM), 100–101
Conjoint couples therapy, 187
Conscious, 180
Conservators, 211
Consta, 197, 200
Constipation, 190
Controlling, 181
Conversion disorder, 141–142
Coprolalia, 128
Correctional psychiatry, 214
Cortisol, 155
Countertransference, 183
Couples therapy, 187
Creutzfeldt-Jakob disease (CJD), 109–110
Criminal law, 210. *See also* Forensic psychiatry
Culture-specific psychoses, 31
Cyclothymic disorder, 43
Cymbalta (duloxetine), 191, 193
CYP450, 190
CYP450 inducers, 190
CYP450 inhibitors, 190–191
Cytochrome P450, 190

D
Da PANICS, 50
Daubert v. Merrell Dow Pharmaceuticals, 213
DBS. *See* Deep brain stimulation (DBS)
DBT. *See* Dialectical behavioral therapy (DBT)
DDAVP. *See* Desmopressin (DDAVP)
Death and dying, 117. *See also* Bereavement
Deconditioning, 184
Deep brain stimulation (DBS), 207
Defense mechanisms, 181–182
Delayed ejaculation, 174

Delayed sleep phase disorder (DPSD), 166
Delirium, 5–6, 99–102
    children, 100
    clinical manifestations, 99–100
    confusion assessment method (CAM), 100–101
    diagnosis, 100–101
    DSM-5 criteria, 101
    epidemiology, 99
    etiology, 99
    head CT, 101
    medication-induced, 99
    other names, 99
    risk factors, 99, 100
    treatment, 101–102
Delirium tremens (DTs), 9, 83
Delusion, 15, 22, 30
Delusional disorder, 30–31
Delusional patient, 18
Delusions of control, 22
Delusions of grandeur, 15, 22
Delusions of guilt, 22
Delusions of persecution, 22
Dementia, 115, 118–119. *See also* Neurocognitive disorders (NCDs)
Demerol (meperidine), 90
Denial, 182
Depakene (valproic acid), 35, 202
Depakote (valproic acid), 35, 202
Dependent personality disorder (DPD), 73, 74–75
Depersonalization/derealization disorder, 135
Depressed patient, 18
Depression, 7. *See also* Major depressive disorder (MDD)
Derealization/depersonalization, 16
Desensitation/imagery rehearsal therapy, 168
Desipramine (norpramin), 194
Desmopressin (DDAVP), 131
Desoxyn (methamphetamine), 87
Desvenlafaxine (Pristiq), 193
Desyrel (trazodone), 161, 193
Developmental history, 13
Dexedrine (dextroamphetamine), 87, 204–205
Dextroamphetamine (Dexedrine), 87, 204–205
Dextromethorphan, 90
Diagnostic testing, 18–19
Dialectical behavioral therapy (DBT), 186
Diazepam (Valium), 203
DID. *See* Dissociative identity disorder (DID)
Difficult patients, 17–18
DIG FAST, 7, 35

Diphenhydramine (Benadryl), 204
Disorders and illnesses
    anxiety disorders, 48–55
    dissociative disorders, 133–137
    eating disorders, 151–157
    geriatric psychiatry, 113–120
    impulse control disorders, 145–149
    mood disorders, 33–45
    neurocognitive disorders, 97–111
    obsessive-compulsive and related disorders, 55–58
    pediatric psychiatry, 121–132
    personality disorders, 63–77
    psychotic disorders, 21–31
    sexual dysfunctions and paraphilic disorders, 171–177
    sleep-wake disorders, 159–169
    somatic symptom and factitious disorders, 139–144
    substance-related and addictive disorders, 79–95
    trauma and stressor-related disorders, 58–61
    treatment. *See* Psychopharmacology; Psychotherapy
Displacement, 181
Disruptive and conduct disorders, 129–130
Disruptive mood dysregulation disorder (DMDD), 44–45
Dissociation, 134
Dissociative amnesia, 134
Dissociative disorders, 133–137
    depersonalization/derealization disorder, 135
    dissociative amnesia, 134
    dissociative identity disorder (DID), 136
    multiple personality disorder, 136
    other specified disorder, 136–137
Dissociative fugue, 134
Dissociative identity disorder (DID), 136
Dissociative trance, 137
Disulfiram (Antabuse), 85
DMDD. *See* Disruptive mood dysregulation disorder (DMDD)
Donepezil (Aricept), 105, 205
Dopamine, 173
Dopamine hypothesis, 26
Down syndrome, 123
Downward drift hypothesis, 26
Doxepin (Sinequan), 161, 194
DPD. *See* Dependent personality disorder (DPD)
DPSD. *See* Delayed sleep phase disorder (DPSD)
Dream interpretation, 183
Dronabinol, 92
Drug interactions, 190–191
Drugs of abuse, 7–8. *See also* Substance-related and addictive disorders

Drunkenness. *See* Alcohol (EtOH)
DTs. *See* Delirium tremens (DTs)
Duloxetine (Cymbalta), 191, 193
Durham rule, 213
Dusky v. United States, 212
Duty to warn, 210
Dysosmias, 160–166
Dysthymia, 42–43
Dystonia, 190, 197

E
Eating disorders, 151–157
　anorexia nervosa, 153–154
　binge-eating disorder, 156–157
　bulimia nervosa, 155–156
Ebstein's anomaly, 201
Echolalia, 128
ECT. *See* Electroconvulsive therapy (ECT)
ED. See Erectile dysfunction (ED)
Effexor (venlafaxine), 192–193
Ego, 180
Elavil (amitriptyline), 161, 194
Elder abuse, 120
Elderly people. *See* Geriatric psychiatry
Electroconvulsive therapy (ECT), 38,
　　41, 206
Elimination disorders, 130–131
Emancipated minors, 211
Emsam transdermal patch, 195
Encopresis, 130–131
Enuresis, 130–131
EPS. *See* Extrapyramidal side effects (EPS)
Erectile disorder, 174, 175
Erectile dysfunction (ED), 173
Erotomanic-type delusion, 30
Escitalopram (Lexapro), 192
Estrogen, 172
Eszopiclone (Lunesta), 161, 204
Ethanol, 82. *See also* Alcohol (EtOH)
EtOH, 81–86. *See also* Alcohol (EtOH)
Examination and diagnosis, 11–19
　diagnosis and classification, 18
　diagnostic testing, 18–19
　difficult patients, 17–18
　history, 12, 13
　interviewing, 12, 17–18
　mental status exam, 14–16
　Mini-Mental State Examination (MMSE), 17

Excoriation disorder, 58
Executive functioning, 180
Exelon (rivastigmine), 105, 205
Exhibitionistic disorder, 177
Extrapyramidal side effects (EPS), 190, 197, 198

F
Factitious disorder, 143–144
Family law, 214
Family psychiatric and medical history, 13
Family therapy, 187
Fanapt (hoperidone), 200
FAS. *See* Fetal alcohol syndrome (FAS)
Faulty assumptions, 185
Female orgasmic disorder, 174, 175
Female sexual interest/arousal disorder, 174, 175
Fetal alcohol syndrome (FAS), 81, 123
Fetishistic disorder, 177
First-generation antipsychotics, 27, 196–198
Five stages of grief, 117
Flat affect, 15
Flight of ideas, 15
Flooding and implosion, 184
Flumazenil, 203
Fluoxetine (Prozac), 156, 190, 191
Fluphenazine (Prolixin), 197
Fluvoxamine (Luvox), 190, 192
Forensic psychiatry, 209–216
　admission to psychiatric hospital, 212
　child and family law, 214
　competence to stand trial, 212
　confidentiality, 210
　correctional psychiatry, 214
　decision making, 211
　decisional capacity, 211
　disability, 212
　emancipated minors, 211
　guardians/conservators, 211
　informed consent, 211
　insanity defense standards, 213
　malingering, 214
　malpractice, 210
　negligence, 210
　not guilty by reason of insanity (NGRI), 213
　risk assessment, 213
　standard of care and malpractice, 210
Four-way couples therapy, 187
Fourteenth Amendment, 212

Fragile X syndrome, 123
Free association, 183
Freud's theories of the mind, 180–181
Frontotemporal degeneration (FTD), 107
Frotteuristic disorder, 177
Frye v. United States, 213
FTD. *See* Frontotemporal degeneration (FTD)
Functional neurological symptom disorder, 141

G

Gabapentin (Neurontin), 202
Gabitril (tiagabine), 202
GAD. *See* Generalized anxiety disorder (GAD)
Galantamine (Razadyne), 105, 205
Gambling disorder, 94–95
Gamma-hydroxybutyrate (GHB), 89
GBMI. *See* Guilty but mentally ill (GBMI)
Gender dysphoria, 176
Gender identity disorder, 176
Generalized anxiety disorder (GAD), 54–55
Genetic syndromes, 123
Genito-pelvic pain/penetration disorder, 174, 176
Geodon (ziprasidone), 200
Geriatric psychiatry, 113–120
  alcohol and medication interactions, 118
  bereavement, 117
  conversion-like presentations, 141
  dementia, 115, 118–119
  elder abuse, 120
  major depression, 114
  medications, 118, 120
  normal aging, 114
  nursing homes, 120
  pseudodementia, 114–115
  restraints, 120
  sexual changes with aging, 172
  sleep disturbance, 119–120
  substance use, 117, 118
GHB. *See* Gamma-hydroxybutyrate (GHB)
Global developmental delay, 123
Grandeur delusion, 15, 22
Grandiose-type delusion, 30
Group therapy, 175, 186
Guardians/conservators, 211
Guilty but mentally ill (GBMI), 213

H

Hair-pulling disorder, 57–58
Halcion (triazolam), 203
Haldol (haloperidol), 101, 119, 197, 199
Hallucinations, 15, 22, 165
Hallucinogens, 48, 91–92
Haloperidol (Haldol), 101, 119, 197, 199
HAM side effects, 190
HD. *See* Huntington's disease (HD)
Heterocyclic antidepressants, 193–194
High-potency antipsychotics, 28, 197
Hinckley, John, 213
History, 12, 13
History of present illness (HPI), 12
Histrionic personality disorder (HPD), 68, 71–72
HIV. *See* Human immunodeficiency virus (HIV)
Hoarding disorder, 57
Hoperidone (Fanapt), 200
HPI. *See* History of present illness (HPI)
Human immunodeficiency virus (HIV), 108
Humor, 181
Huntington's disease (HD), 108–109
Hydroxyzine (Atarax), 204
Hyperprolactinemia, 190, 197
Hypersomnias, 160
Hypersomnolence disorder, 161–162
Hypertensive crisis, 9, 190, 195
Hyperthyroidism, 103
Hypnagogic hallucination, 165
Hypnopompic hallucination, 165
Hypokinesia, 13
Hypomanic episode, 35
Hypothyroidism, 103

I

ICU psychosis, 99, 100
ID. *See* Intellectual disability (ID)
Id, 180
Ideas of reference, 22
Illegal drugs. *See* Substance-related and addictive disorders
Illness anxiety disorder, 142
Illusions, 16, 22
IM-Vivitrol (naltrexone), 85
Imagery rehearsal therapy (IRT), 168
Imipramine (Tofranil), 131, 194
Impotence, 173

Impulse control disorders, 145–149
 intermittent explosive disorder, 145–147
 kleptomania, 147–148
 pyromania, 148
IMPULSIVE, 71
Inappropriate affect, 14
Informed consent, 211
Inhalants, 93
Insanity, 213
Insanity Defense Reform Act, 213
Insanity defense standards, 213
Insomnia disorder, 160–161
Intellectual disability (ID), 122–123
Intellectualization, 182
Intelligence quotient (IQ), 18, 19
Intermittent explosive disorder, 145–147
Interpersonal therapy, 183
Interviewing, 12, 17–18
Invega (paliperidone), 197, 200
Involuntary admission to psychiatric hospital, 212
IQ. See Intelligence quotient (IQ)
Irresistible impulse, 213
Irritability, 35
IRT. See Imagery rehearsal therapy (IRT)
Isocarboxazid (Marplan), 195
Isolation of affect, 182
Isoniazid, 206

J

Jealous-type delusion, 31
Jet lag disorder, 166

K

K-ABC. See Kaufman Assessment Battery for Children (K-ABC)
Kaufman Assessment Battery for Children (K-ABC), 122
Ketamine, 88
Kleptomania, 147–148
Klonopin (clonazepam), 107, 203
Koro, 31
Korsakoff syndrome, 84, 86
Kübler-Ross, Elisabeth, 117

L

Labile affect, 14
Lamotrigine (Lamictal), 202
Language disorder, 124
Latuda (lurasidone), 200
LBD. See Lewy body disease (LBD)
Learning disorder, 123–124
Learning theory, 184
Legal issues, 210. See also Forensic psychiatry
Leukocytosis, 201
Levodopa-carbidopa, 107, 109
Lewy body disease (LBD), 106–107
Lexapro (escitalopram), 192
Light therapy, 207
Lithium, 41, 200–201
Lithium toxicity, 9
Lorazepam (Ativan), 203
Loosening of associations, 15
Low-potency antipsychotics, 28, 196–197
Loxapine (Loxitane), 197
LSD. See Lysergic acid diethylamide (LSD)
LSD flashback, 92
Lunesta (eszopiclone), 161, 204
Lurasidone (Latuda), 200
Luvox (fluvoxamine), 190, 192
Lyrica (pregabalin), 202
Lysergic acid diethylamide (LSD), 8, 91

M

Major depressive disorder (MDD), 34, 36–40
 anorexia nervosa, 154
 antidepressant medication, 37–38
 bereavement-associated depression, 117
 course and prognosis, 37
 diagnosis, 34, 36
 ECT, 38
 epidemiology, 36
 etiology, 37
 hospitalization, 38
 psychotherapy, 38
 sleep problems, 36
 treatment, 37–38
Major depressive episode, 34
Major neurocognitive disorders (NCDs), 102, 103
Male hypoactive sexual desire disorder, 174, 175
Malingering, 144, 214
Malpractice, 210
Mania, 7
Manic-depression, 40
Manic episode, 34–35

MAOIs. *See* Monamine oxidase inhibitors (MAOIs)

Marijuana, 81, 92. *See also* Cannabis

Marplan (isocarboxazid), 195

MDD. *See* Major depressive disorder (MDD)

Medical conditions. *See* Disorders and illnesses

Medical history, 13

Medication. *See* Psychopharmacology

Medication-induced bipolar disorder, 36

Medication-induced delirium, 99

Medication-induced depressive disorder, 36

Medication-induced psychotic disorder, 23

Melatonin, 107

Mellaril (thioridazine), 197

Memantine (Namenda), 205

Memory cards. *See* Pocket cards

Mental disability, 212

Mental impairment, 212

Mental retardation, 122–123

Mental status exam, 5, 14–16

Meperidine (Demerol), 90

Mescaline, 91

Metabolic encephalopathy, 99

Metabolic syndrome, 28, 200

Meth mouth, 88

Methadone, 91

Methamphetamine (Desoxyn), 87

Methylphenidate (Ritalin), 87, 115, 205

Midazolam (Versed), 203

Midpotency antipsychotics, 197

Mild neurocognitive disorders (NCDs), 102, 103

Mini-Cog, 103

Mini-Mental State Examination (MMSE), 6, 17, 104

Minnesota Multiphasic Personality Inventory (MMPI-2), 18, 19

Mirtazapine (Remeron), 115, 193

Mixed-type delusion, 31

MMPI-2. *See* Minnesota Multiphasic Personality Inventory (MMPI-2)

MMSE. *See* Mini-Mental State Examination (MMSE)

M'Naghten rule, 213

Moban (molindone), 197

Modafinil (Provigil), 205

Molindone (Moban), 197

Monamine oxidase inhibitors (MAOIs), 37–38, 49

Monoamine oxidase inhibitors (MAOIs), 195

Mood, 34

Mood disorders, 33–45

   bereavement, 40

   bipolar disorders, 40–42

   cyclothymic disorder, 43

   differential diagnosis, 35–36

   disruptive mood dysregulation disorder (DMDD), 44–45

   dysthymia, 42–43

   major depressive disorder (MDD), 34, 36–40

   mood episodes, 34–35

   other disorders, 45

   persistent depressive disorder, 42–43

   premenstrual dysphoric disorder, 43–44

   specifiers for depressive disorders, 39–40

   substance/medication-induced disorders, 36

Mood episodes, 34–35

Mood stabilizers, 200–201

Morphine, 90

Multiple personality disorder, 136

Münchhausen syndrome, 143

Münchhausen syndrome by proxy, 143

N

Naloxone, 90

Naltrexone (Revia), 85, 91

Namenda (memantine), 205

Narcissistic personality disorder (NPD), 68, 72–73

Narcolepsy, 165

Narcoleptic cataplexy, 165

Nardil (phenelzine), 195

Navane (thiothixene), 197

NCDs. *See* Neurocognitive disorders (NCDs)

Nefazodone (Serzone), 193

Negative reinforcement, 184

Negative thoughts, 185

Neglect of child, 132

Negligence, 210

Neologisms, 15

Neurocognitive disorders (NCDs), 97–111

   Alzheimer's disease (AD), 104–105

   Creutzfeldt-Jakob disease (CJD), 109–110

   delirium, 99–102

   dementia, 115, 118–119

   frontotemporal degeneration (FTD), 107

   HIV infection, 108

   Huntington's disease (HD), 108–109

   Lewy body disease (LBD), 106–107

   major NCDs, 102, 103

   mild NCDs, 102, 103

   MMSE, 6, 17, 104

   normal pressure hydrocephalus (NPH), 110–111

Neurocognitive disorders (NCDs) (*Continued*)
  Parkinson's disease (PD), 109
  prion disease, 109–110
  vascular disease (vascular cognitive impairment),
    105–106
Neurofibrillary tangles, 105
Neuroleptic malignant syndrome (NMS), 9, 28, 198.
    See also Tardive dyskinesia (TD)
Neurontin (gabapentin), 202
Neurotic defenses, 181–182
NGRI. *See* Not guilty by reason of insanity (NGRI)
Nicotine, 8, 94
Nicotine replacement therapy (NRT), 94
Nifedipine, 206
Nightmare disorder, 168
NMDA (glutamate) receptor antagonist, 205
NMS. *See* Neuroleptic malignant syndrome (NMS)
Non-REM sleep arousal disorders, 166–167
Nonbizarre delusion, 22
Norepinephrine-dopamine reuptake inhibitors, 193
Normal grief, 117
Normal pressure hydrocephalus (NPH), 110–111
Norpramin (desipramine), 194
Nortriptyline (Pamelor, Aventyl), 194
Not guilty by reason of insanity (NGRI), 213
NPD. *See* Narcissistic personality disorder (NPD)
NPH. *See* Normal pressure hydrocephalus (NPH)
NREM sleep, 160
NRT. *See* Nicotine replacement therapy (NRT)
Nursing homes, 120

O
OBEDIENT, 75
Objective personality assessment tests, 19
Obsessive-compulsive and related disorders, 55–58
  body dysmorphic disorder, 56
  excoriation disorder, 58
  hair-pulling disorder, 57–58
  hoarding disorder, 57
  obsessive-compulsive disorder (OCD), 55–56
  skin-picking disorder, 58
  trichotillomania, 57–58
Obsessive-compulsive disorder (OCD), 55–56
Obsessive-compulsive personality disorder (OCPD),
    56, 68, 75–76
Obstructive sleep apnea hypopnea, 162–163
OCD. *See* Obsessive-compulsive disorder (OCD)
OCPD. *See* Obsessive-compulsive personality disorder
    (OCPD)

ODD. *See* Oppositional defiant disorder (ODD)
Olanzapine (Zyprexa), 119, 200
Older persons. *See* Geriatric psychiatry
Olfactory hallucination, 22
On Death and Dying (Kübler-Ross), 117
Open-ended questions, 12
Operant conditioning, 184
Opioids, 8, 48, 81, 90–91
Oppositional defiant disorder (ODD), 129
Orap (pimozile), 197
Orgasm, 172
Other specified dissociative disorder,
    136–137
Other specified personality disorder, 76
Out-of-body experience (depersonalization), 135
Overview. *See* Disorders and illnesses
Oxazepam (Serax), 203
Oxcarbazepine (Trileptal), 202

P
Pain attack, 49–50
Paliperidone (Invega), 197, 200
Pamelor (nortriptyline), 194
Panic disorder, 50
Paranoid delusion, 15, 22
Paranoid personality disorder (PPD), 65–66
Paraphilic disorders, 176–177
Parasomnias, 166–169
Parkinsonism, 190, 197
Parkinson's disease (PD), 109
Parnate (tranylcypromine), 195
Paroxetine (Paxil), 190, 192
Past psychiatric history, 13
Patient rights, 3
Paxil (paroxetine), 190, 192
PCP. *See* Phencyclidine (PCP)
PD. *See* Parkinson's disease (PD)
Pediatric psychiatry, 121–132
  ADHD, 125–126
  autism spectrum disorder (ASD), 126–127
  bed-wetting, 130–131
  child abuse, 131–132
  communication disorders, 124
  conduct disorder, 129–130
  delirium, 100
  disruptive and conduct disorders, 129–130
  elimination disorders, 130–131
  genetic syndromes, 123
  global developmental delay, 123

Pediatric psychiatry (*Continued*)
  information-gathering methods, 122
  intellectual disability (ID), 122–123
  mental retardation, 122–123
  neglect, 132
  oppositional defiant disorder (ODD), 129
  psychiatric examination, 122
  psychological abuse, 132
  specific learning disorder, 123–124
  tic disorders, 128–129
  Tourette's disorder, 128–129
Pedophilic disorder, 177
Pentobarbital, 204
Perceptual disturbances, 15–16, 22
Performance anxiety, 52
Periodic leg movements (PLMs), 119
Perphenazine (Trilafon), 197
Persecutory-type delusion, 30
Persistent depressive disorder, 42–43
Persistent motor or vocal tic disorder, 129
Personality, 64
Personality assessment tests, 19
Personality change due to another medical condition, 76
Personality disorder, 63–77
  antisocial, 68, 69–70
  avoidant, 73–74
  borderline, 68, 70–71
  CAPRI, 64
  clusters, 64
  dependent, 73, 74–75
  diagnosis and DSM-5 criteria, 64
  etiology, 64
  histrionic, 68, 71–72
  narcissistic, 68, 72–73
  obsessive-compulsive, 73, 75–76
  other specified, 76
  paranoid, 65–66
  personality change due to another medical
    condition, 76
  schizoid, 65, 66–67
  schizotypal, 65, 67–68
  treatment, 65
  unspecified, 76
Pharmacologic treatment. *See* Psychopharmacology
Phencyclidine (PCP), 81, 88–89
Phenelzine (Nardil), 195
Phenobarbital, 204
Phobia, 51
Phonological disorder, 124

Phosphodiesterase-5 inhibitors, 175
Phototherapy, 207
Pimozile (Orap), 197
Play therapy, 122
PLMs. *See* Periodic leg movements (PLMs)
Pocket cards
  acute dystonia, 9
  delirium, 5–6
  delirium tremens (DTs), 9
  depression, 7
  drugs of abuse, 7–8
  lithium toxicity, 9
  mania, 7
  mental status exam, 5
  Mini-Mental State Examination (MMSE), 6
  neuroleptic malignant syndrome (NMS), 9
  psychiatric emergencies, 9
  serotonin syndrome, 9
  suicide risk, 7
  tricyclic antidepressant (TCA) toxicity, 9
  tyramine reaction/hypertensive crisis, 9
Polysomnography, 163
Positive reinforcement, 184
Postpartum period, 38
Posttraumatic stress disorder (PTSD), 59–60
PPD. *See* Paranoid personality disorder (PPD)
Prader-Willi syndrome, 123
Pragmatic communication disorder, 124
Prazosin, 168
Preconscious, 180
Pregabalin (Lyrica), 202
Premature ejaculation, 174, 175–176
Premenstrual dysphoric disorder, 43–44
Presenting patient information, 3–4
Pressured speech, 14
Prion disease, 109–110
Pristiq (desvenlafaxine), 193
Procainamide, 206
Projection, 182
Projective assessment tests, 19
Prolixin (fluphenazine), 197
Propranolol, 49, 204
Proverb testing, 18
Provigil (modafinil), 205
Provisional tic disorder, 129
Prozac (fluoxetine), 156, 190, 191
Pseudodementia, 114–115
Pseudoephedrine, 88
Psilocybin, 91

Psychiatric disorders. *See* Disorders and illnesses
Psychiatric emergencies, 9
Psychiatric history, 12, 13
Psychiatry clerkship, 2
Psychoanalysis, 182–183
Psychoanalytically oriented psychotherapy, 183
Psychodynamic psychotherapy, 49
Psychological abuse, 132
Psychomotor retardation, 13
Psychopharmacology, 189–207
    anticonvulsants, 201–202
    antidepressants, 191–194, 195–196
    antipsychotics, 196–200
    anxiolytics/hypnotics, 202–204
    cognitive enhancers, 205
    drug interactions, 190–191
    medications causing psychiatric symptoms, 205–206
    monoamine oxidase inhibitors (MAOIs), 195
    mood stabilizers, 200–201
    psychostimulants, 204–205
    side effects, 190–191
Psychosis, 22–23
Psychostimulants, 204–205
Psychotherapy, 38, 49, 179–187
    behavioral therapy, 184
    cognitive-behavioral therapy (CBT), 185
    cognitive therapy, 185
    couples therapy, 187
    defense mechanisms, 181–182
    dialectical behavioral therapy (DBT), 186
    family therapy, 187
    Freud's theories of the mind, 180–181
    group therapy, 186
    immature defenses, 182
    learning theory, 184
    neurotic defenses, 181–182
    psychoanalysis, 182–183
Psychotic disorder due to another medical condition, 23
Psychotic disorders, 21–31
    brief psychotic disorder, 30
    culture-specific psychoses, 31
    delusional disorder, 30–31
    distinguishing features, 31
    prognosis, 31
    psychosis, 22–23
    schizoaffective disorder, 29
    schizophrenia, 23–29
    schizophreniform disorder, 29
    time course, 31

PTSD. *See* Posttraumatic stress disorder (PTSD)
Punitive damages, 210
Pyromania, 148

Q
Quetiapine (Seroquel), 107, 109, 119, 200
Quick reference. *See* Pocket cards
Quinidine, 206

R
Ramelteon (Rozerem), 204
Rapid cycling, 40
Rationalization, 182
Razadyne (galantamine), 105, 205
Reaction formation, 182
Reagan assassination attempt, 213
Recurrent major depressive episodes with hypomania, 41
RED DANES, 88
Refeeding syndrome, 154
Reference delusion, 15
Regression, 72, 182
Religious delusion, 15
REM sleep, 160, 161
REM sleep behavior disorder, 168–169
Remeron (mirtazapine), 115, 193
Repetitive transcranial magnetic stimulation (rTMS), 207
Repression, 182
Restless legs syndrome, 169
Restoril (temazepam), 203
Restricting-type anorexia, 153
Revia (naltrexone), 85, 91
Risperidone (Risperdal), 119, 197, 200
Ritalin (methylphenidate), 87, 115, 205
Rivastigmine (Exelon), 105, 205
Rorschach test, 19
Rosa's law, 122
Rotatory nystagmus, 88
Rozerem (Ramelteon), 204
rTMS. *See* Repetitive transcranial magnetic stimulation (rTMS)
Russell's sign, 155

S
SAD PERSONS, 7
Saphris (asenapine), 200
Schizoaffective disorder, 29

Schizoid personality disorder, 65, 66–67
Schizophrenia, 23–29
    5 A's, 24
    delusional disorder, contrasted, 30
    dopamine hypothesis, 26
    downward drift, 26
    DSM-5 criteria, 24
    epidemiology, 26
    genetic component, 27
    neurotransmitter abnormalities, 27
    overview, 30
    pathophysiology, 26
    phases, 24
    positive, negative, and cognitive symptoms, 24
    prognostic factors, 27
    psychiatric exam, 25–26
    side effects of medication, 28–29
    treatment, 27–29
Schizophreniform disorder, 29
Schizotypal personality disorder, 65, 67–68
Seasonal affective disorder, 40, 207
Second-generation antipsychotics, 28, 199–200
Secondary amines, 194
Sedative-hypnotics, 48, 81, 89–90
Selective mutism, 52–53
Selective serotonin reuptake inhibitors (SSRIs), 38,
        191–192
Selegiline, 195
Senile plaques, 105
Separation anxiety disorder, 53
Serax (oxazepam), 203
Seroquel (quetiapine), 107, 109, 119, 200
Serotonin, 173
Serotonin-norepinephrine reuptake inhibitors (SNRIs),
        192–193
Serotonin receptor antagonists and agonists, 193
Serotonin syndrome, 9, 38, 190, 192, 195
Sertraline (Zoloft), 191, 192
Serzone (nefazodone), 193
Sex therapy, 174
Sexual dysfunctions and paraphilic disorders, 171–177
    analytically oriented (psychodynamic)
        psychotherapy, 175
    cognitive-behavioral therapy, 175
    delayed ejaculation, 174
    differential diagnosis, 172–173
    erectile disorder, 174, 175
    female orgasmic disorder, 174, 175
    female sexual interest/arousal disorder, 174, 175

    gender dysphoria, 176
    genito-pelvic pain/penetration disorder, 174, 176
    group therapy, 175
    hypnosis, 175
    male hypoactive sexual desire disorder, 174, 175
    mechanical therapies, 175–176
    paraphilias, 176–177
    pharmacologic treatment, 175
    premature ejaculation, 174, 175–176
    sex therapy, 174
    sexual changes with aging, 172
    sexual response cycle, 172
Sexual masochism disorder, 177
Sexual response cycle, 172
Shelf examination, 4
Shift-work disorder (SWD), 166
Shoplifting, 147–148
SIG E. CAPS, 7, 34
Sildenafil, 175
Simple grief, 40
Sinequan (doxepin), 161, 194
Sixth Amendment, 212
Skin-picking disorder, 58
Sleep apnea, 162–163
Sleep disturbance, 119–120
Sleep-related hypoventilation, 163–164
Sleep terrors, 167–168
Sleep-wake disorders, 159–169
    central sleep apnea, 163
    circadian rhythm sleep wake disorders, 165–166
    dysosmias, 160–166
    hypersomnolence disorder, 161–162
    insomnia disorder, 160–161
    narcolepsy, 165
    nightmare disorder, 168
    non-REM sleep arousal disorders, 166–167
    normal sleep-wake cycle, 160
    obstructive sleep apnea hypopnea, 162–163
    parasomnias, 166–169
    REM sleep behavior disorder, 168–169
    restless legs syndrome, 169
    sleep history, 160
    sleep-related hypoventilation, 163–164
    sleep terrors, 167–168
    sleepwalking, 167
Sleepwalking, 167
SNRIs. See Serotonin-norepinephrine reuptake
        inhibitors (SNRIs)
Social anxiety disorder, 51–52

Social communication disorder, 124
Social history, 13
Social phobia, 51–52
Social and/or Occupational Dysfunction (SOD), 48
Somatic delusion, 15, 22, 30
Somatic symptom and factitious disorders, 139–144
   conversion disorder, 141–142
   distinguishing features, 144
   factitious disorder, 143–144
   illness anxiety disorder, 142
   malingering, 144
   psychological factors affecting other conditions, 142–143
   somatic symptom disorder, 140–141, 144
Somatic symptom disorder, 140–141, 144
Sonata (zaleplon), 89, 161, 204
Special K (ketamine), 88
Specific learning disorder, 123–124
Specific phobias, 51–52
Speech sound disorder, 124
Splitting, 182
Spousal abuse, 82
Squeeze technique, 175
SSRIs. *See* Selective serotonin reuptake inhibitors (SSRIs)
St. John's wort, 190
Standard of care, 210
Stelazine (trifluoperazine), 197
Steroids, 206
Stevens-Johnson syndrome, 201, 202
Stimulants, 48
Stop-start technique, 176
Strattera (atomoxetine), 205
Stressor-related disorders, 58–61
Stroke patients, 36
Stuttering, 124
Sublimation, 181
Substance history, 13
Substance-induced bipolar disorder, 36
Substance-induced depressive disorder, 36
Substance/medication-induced psychotic disorder, 23
Substance-related and addictive disorders, 7–8, 79–95
   acute intoxication and withdrawal, 80
   alcohol (EtOH), 81–86
   amphetamines, 87–88
   caffeine, 93–94
   cocaine, 87
   detection of substance use, 81
   diagnosis and DSM-5 criteria, 80

   epidemiology, 80
   gambling disorder, 94–95
   geriatric patients, 117, 118
   hallucinogens, 91–92
   inhalants, 93
   marijuana, 92
   nicotine, 94
   opioids, 90–91
   phencyclidine (PCP), 88–89
   psychiatric symptoms, 80
   sedative-hypnotics, 89–90
   treatment, 81
Suicide risk, 7
Superego, 180
Supportive psychotherapy, 183
Suppression, 181
Suprachiasmic nucleus (SCN), 166
SWD. *See* Shift-work disorder (SWD)
Systematic desensitization, 184

T
Tactile hallucination, 22
Tangentiality, 15
Tarasoff duty, 210
Tarasoff rule, 18
Tardive dyskinesia (TD), 28, 190, 198
TAT. *See* Thematic apperception test (TAT)
TCA overdose, 194
TCA toxicity. *See* Tricyclic antidepressant (TCA) toxicity
TCAs. *See* Tricyclic antidepressants (TCAs)
TD. *See* Tardive dyskinesia (TD)
Team player, 3
Tegretol (carbamazepine), 190, 201
Temazepam (Restoril), 203
Tertiary amines, 194
Testosterone, 173
Tetracyclic antidepressants, 194
Tetracycline, 206
Tetrahydrocannabinol (THC), 92
THC. *See* Tetrahydrocannabinol (THC)
Thematic apperception test (TAT), 19
Therapeutic alliance, 183
Thioridazine (Mellaril), 197
Thiothixene (Navane), 197
Thorazine (chlorpromazine), 196–197
Thought blocking, 15
Thought broadcasting, 15, 22

Thought content, 15
Thought insertion, 22
Thought process, 15
Thyroid dysfunction, 103
Tiagabine (Gabitril), 202
Tic disorders, 128–129
Tics, 128
Tobacco, 48, 190
Tofranil (imipramine), 131, 194
Token economy, 184
Topamax (topiramate), 85, 202
Topiramate (Topamax), 85, 202
TORCH, 123
Tourette's disorder, 128–129
Toxic encephalopathy, 99
Transference, 183
Transgendered persons, 176
Transsexuality, 176
Transvestic disorder, 177
Tranylcypromine (Parnate), 195
TRAUMA, 60
Trauma and stressor-related disorders
    acute stress disorder, 59
    adjustment disorder, 60–61
    posttraumatic stress disorder (PTSD), 59–60
Trazodone (Desyrel), 161, 193
Treatment. See Psychopharmacology; Psychotherapy
Triangles, 187
Triazolam (Halcion), 203
Trichotillomania, 57–58
Tricyclic antidepressant (TCA) toxicity, 9
Tricyclic antidepressants (TCAs), 37, 49, 194
Trifluoperazine (Stelazine), 197
Trilafon (Perphenazine), 197
Trileptal (oxcarbazepine), 202
Typical antipsychotics, 27, 196–198
Tyramine reaction/hypertensive crisis, 9

U
Unconscious, 180
Undoing, 182
Unspecified personality disorder, 76

V
VALEUMS, 100
Valium (diazepam), 203

Valproic acid (Depakote, Depakene), 35, 202
Varenicline (Chantix), 94
Vascular cognitive impairment, 105–106
Vascular disease, 105–106
Venlafaxine (Effexor), 192–193
Verapamil, 206
Versed (midazolam), 203
Violent patient, 17–18
Visual hallucination, 22
Vocal tics, 128
Voluntary admission to psychiatric hospital, 212
Volunteering, 3
Voyeuristic disorder, 177

W
WAIS. See Wechsler Adult Intelligence Scale (WAIS)
Wards, how to behave, 2–4
Wechsler Adult Intelligence Scale (WAIS), 18
Wechsler Intelligence Scale for Children (WISC), 19
Wechsler Intelligence Scale for Children-Revised (WISC-R), 122
Wellbutrin. See Bupropion (Wellbutrin, Zyban)
Wernicke's encephalopathy, 82, 86
WISC. See Wechsler Intelligence Scale for Children (WISC)
WISC-R. See Wechsler Intelligence Scale for Children-Revised (WISC-R)
Word salad, 15
Worry WARTS, 54

X
Xanax (alprazolam), 203

Z
Zaleplon (Sonata), 89, 161, 204
Ziprasidone (Geodon), 200
Zoloft (sertraline), 191, 192
Zolpidem (Ambien), 89, 161, 204
Zyban. See Bupropion (Wellbutrin, Zyban)
Zyprexa (olanzapine), 119, 200